The joy of HOSPITAL CLOWNING

Making a Difference With
Love and Laughter

Authors:
Anita Thies
Kathy Piatt
Tammy Miller

Illustrator:
Bill Moore

Cover Design:
David Maser

Wishing you joy, love, and laughter — Anita Thies

Copyright 2000 ©
Revised Edition Copyright 2003 ©
by Lighthearted Press
ISBN # 0-9701379-1-5
Library of Congress Control Number: 2003092914

Published by
Lighthearted Press
761 Cornwall Rd.
State College, PA 16803

Dedications

From Anita to my mother Virginia Rose Boyd Hawickhorst Gosney who brought love and laughter to so many and is now with the Lord, and to my loving and supportive husband Jim and son Bill.

From Kathy to Bud – great clown, greater mentor and most of all - the greatest of fathers...and to my soul mate John.

From Tammy to my daughters, Tiffany and Lacey, my partner in comedy, Charlie, and my mother, Ruth for supporting all my zany ideas and sharing the laughter.

From Bill to Carol, my loving and supportive wife, who has been my partner in marriage, in life, and in ministry.

Special Appreciation

To Richard Snowberg for teaching us all about caring clowning and for his continuing support 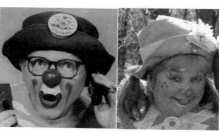 To Shobhana "Shobi Dobi" Schwebke whose life and newsletter reflect the heart of caring clowning

To David Maser for his generous time, talent and spirit in designing the cover for this edition.

To all the clowns who contributed through picture, word and prayer to this edition.

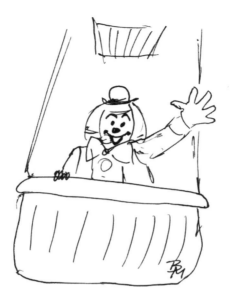

Start Your Journey With Joy

This book came from a clown-like stirring in our hearts
to offer joy and hope.   To be of service.
To give what we have and to share a laugh
– which is what clowning is all about.

We longed for simple, practical clarity.
To realize the importance of humor
and its healing potential.
The great joy of hospital clowning
is that there is SO much
to say, to learn and to celebrate.

Our goal is to offer an overview
of basic thoughts and principles of clowning in hospitals.
We hope to encourage, enlighten and guide.

May you find for yourself in these pages
some of the joy, hope and laughter
that your clown character gives so caringly to others.

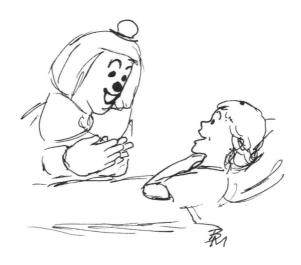

I serve with joy: I clown

"God has brought me joy and laughter;
Whoever hears of this will laugh with me"
Genesis 21: 6

"There is not much laughter
in medicine,
but there is much medicine
in laughter"

—Bud "Buddy the Clown" Salloum
Co-Founder,
Edmonton, Canada Caring Clowns
(shown at right)

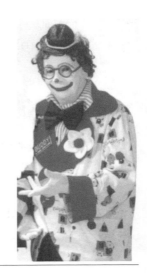

⊓⊓⊓ Of Contents

Chapter 1
Why Be a Hospital Clown?

You Can Make a Difference

They don't want to be here,

alone in an unfamiliar bed.

Yet this is their home for now,

And you can ask to enter.

> *They don't know you and weren't expecting you.*
>
> *They don't know what you'll do*
>
> *or what to make of you.*
>
> *And you can't know what they need most.*

They may be scared or lonely, bored or hurting.

They may be all of that and more.

They may have only enough energy

to watch you with their eyes.

> *They may not want to talk*
>
> *or they may want a listener.*
>
> *They may long to laugh*
>
> *and have their spirits lightened.*
>
> *They may need to cry*
>
> *and have their hand held.*

Perhaps a nurse can brief you first.

But you may not know much in advance.

What you do know

is that you are a privileged visitor.

Someone who can bring

a new way of relating to them.

> *You are a caring clown*
>
> *and you train for this moment.*
>
> *Knowing what you give can be like light.*

Lifting a spirit,

Showing things in a new way.

Focusing thoughts away from darkness.

Warming a soul.

> *It is not always that way, of course.*
>
> *Sometimes things go poorly.*
>
> *Often you never know*
>
> *the difference you have made.*

But there are times that seem to say

this is where you are needed . . .

as clown and caring person.

This is where you can open your heart

to serve and share God's love. — *By Anita Thies*

The Healing Power of Laughter and Caring

There *is* a healing power in laughter.

Over the past three decades, researchers from many areas of study, including medicine and psychology, have become interested in the scientific benefits of laughter. Today a credit selective course in "The Medicine of Laughter" is offered at a leading medical school—the Washington University School of Medicine in St. Louis.

Hooray for endorphins!

Studies have shown that laughter can lower blood pressure and release healthy endorphins, those chemicals in the brain that can ease pain and make you feel better.

Good for the heart

One such study in a hospital setting involved Janet "Jelly Bean" Tucker. The research indicated a rise in the patient's blood pressure as a clown entered the room (presumably from the patient seeing a non-traditional health practitioner) but after the clown left the room, the patient's blood pressure dropped to lower than it was before the clown appeared.

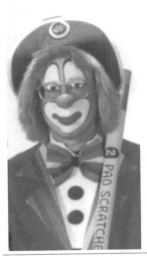

A doctor's perspective

"Not many things are more rewarding and challenging than clowning in a hospital environment.

"Laughter is medicine -- with no co-pay required.

"Humor promotes holistic healing."

—Dr. John Piatt, a family practice physician who has attended Clown Camp® as "Kernel" the Clown *(left)*.

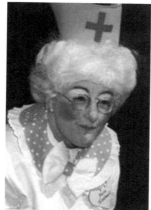
Patty Wooten as
Nurse Kindheart

Nursing Wisdom

National humorist, clown and nurse Patty Wooten says in her book *Compassionate Laughter*:

"*Humor and laughter can foster a positive and hopeful attitude. We are less likely to succumb to feelings of depression and helplessness if we are able to laugh at what is troubling us.*

"*Humor gives us a sense of perspective on our problems. Laughter provides an opportunity for the release of those uncomfortable emotions which, if held inside, may create biochemical changes that are harmful to the body.*" [1]

Leslie Gibson, RN, author of
Laughter, The Universal Language,
observes that:

**"Caring clowns
are opening the doors
for patients to experience
the healing power of humor."**

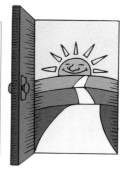

A chaplain speaks of healing

The healing potential of the hospital clown has been observed by the Rev. George Burn, Director of Pastoral Care at Centre Community Hospital (PA):

"Hospitals tend to be somber places and people tend to be focused on the sadness and struggles of their journeys.

"It is healing to have, even for a moment, the ability to remove yourself from that preoccupation and to find laughter once again in the midst of your darkness." [2]

> *"We have a healing power that works in many ways, maybe not to cure, but to lessen the pain."*
> —Don "Homer The Clown" Burda

Merry Heart Medicine

Notes Desi "Dizzy" Payne, who developed the Merry Heart Medicine Program at Ottumwa (Iowa) Regional Health Center, "My slogan is from Proverbs 17:22 : *A merry heart doeth good like a medicine.* Based on this, I give a good dose of medicine every time I'm at the hospital."

The very act of laughing is beneficial. "One of the greatest parts about laughter is that your body doesn't know you are faking it sometimes, " says Tammy Miller, *(right),* author of *The Lighter Side of Breast Cancer Recovery.* "It will still release endorphins that help us heal and cope with situations."

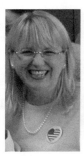

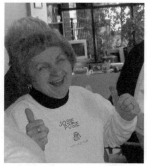

Jo "Josie Posie" Moore of the Happy Valley Alley, World Clown Association, joins with gusto in the group's belly laugh time.

Mark Twain to Emmett Kelly

The benefits of humor were observed many years ago. Mark Twain once said, *"Against the assault of laughter, nothing can stand."*

When Emmett Kelly performed, he noted, *"By laughing at me, they really laugh at themselves, and realizing that they have done this gives them a sort of spiritual second wind for going back into the battle of life."*

> *"Our patients have remarked that just seeing these clowns makes them smile in a time when smiles can be hard to come by."*
> --Rosemarie Tucci, RN, MSN, AOCN, Administrator, Main Line Health Community (PA) Clinical Oncology Program, speaking of the Bumper "T" Caring Clowns.

Humor Therapy

In the 1970s, Norman Cousins' work *Anatomy of an Illness* [3] sparked popular interest in the physiological effects of laughter. Today "humor therapy" is underway in such diverse fields as pediatrics, oncology, geriatrics and psychology and in hospitals such as Rochester General Hospital in New York and Morton Plant Mease Healthcare in Florida.

Arts and Health Outreach Initiative (AHOI)

The convergence between the arts and healing is drawing increased attention from researchers and educators.

"There is an increasing body of empirical research that demonstrates distinct health benefits from participation in live arts experiences," says Ermyn King, Coordinator of the Arts and Health Outreach Initiative (AHOI) at Penn State University.

This innovative initiative at one of the nation's leading land-grant universities is bringing together four principal Penn State partners (including the College of Medicine) to stimulate cutting-edge, interdisciplinary research and programs in the intersection of arts and health. (For more on AHOI see p. 70)

The inspiration of Christopher Reeve

While bringing laughter is rarely a matter of life and death, connecting with a patient's inner spirit through laughter can be profound. Aviva "DR HuggaBubbe" Gorstein *(right)* of the Bumper "T" Caring Clowns says their clown team is inspired by reports of what happened when actor Robin Williams first visited his paralyzed friend Christopher Reeve and prompted him to laugh.

"Robin didn't come to visit a 'spinal cord' or 'nerve endings' but the essence of who Christopher Reeve is," she says, "and when Christopher realized that, he understood that even though his body might be compromised, his mind and his spirit were alive and well. That essence of what a caring clown can be is what motivates us to enter a patient's room with nothing on the agenda but to help rekindle that special spirit that is often hidden inside a hospital gown."

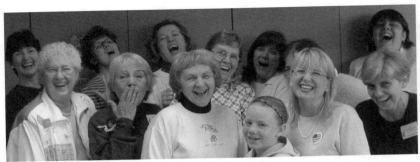

Treating themselves to a healthy workout, members of the Happy Valley Alley of the World Clown Association in State College, PA schedule a time of "belly laughing" at each business meeting, adding one second to the laugh time every month. A high achieving group, at last laugh, they were up to 43 seconds of belly laughing at a time.

The value, the worth and the power of mirth

"The value, the worth, and the power of mirth
Can help each of us to get through,
When the going is rough and incredibly tough,
And even the sunshine looks blue.
For once you give in to a chuckle or grin,
Your spirits just natur'lly lift,
And life is worthwhile each time that you smile,
For a laugh is a God-given gift."
—author unknown, quoted in *The Caring Clowns: How Humor Smiles and Laughter Overcome Pain; Suffering and Loneliness* (Richard Snowberg)[4]

The gift that keeps on giving

Why be a hospital clown? Because with the healing gift of laughter and caring, you can make a difference in the life of a child or an adult; a patient, caregiver, or friend.

The wonderful joy for you is that by giving the gift, you too receive it back many times over. In the words of Patch Adams, M.D.:

"Giving to others is really a gigantic gift to yourself."

Chapter 2
Is Hospital Clowning for You?

Know Yourself

There are many possibilities for clowns in hospitals. Yet not every clown with a caring heart is comfortable in or suited for all hospital situations.

Know what you're looking for

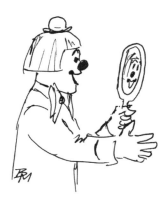

You need to know who you are and what you are looking for from the situation.

If you are a clown who really wants laughter from a large crowd, then hospital clowning is not for you.

A hospital room or ward filled with ill patients presents a completely different situation for a clown than a group of healthy participating people.

Don't expect responses

In the hospital, patients are sometimes unable to respond to you and your humor. Sometimes a response will come back very quietly and sometimes not at all.

The patient ALWAYS comes first

In hospital clowning, the needs of the patient and audience always come before the needs of the performer.

As Richard "Snowflake" Snowberg notes:
"Caring clowns are more interested in assisting people to forget their pains and problems than in generating applause or even laughter." [5]

Why Caring Clowning is a difficult specialty

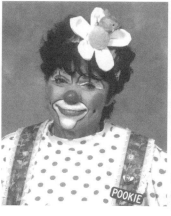

"Caring Clowning is one of the most difficult specialties," says Carole "Pookie" Johnson, *(left)*, a nationally known Caring Clown and Instructor.

"That's because you have to be prepared to meet many different needs, not just of the patients but also of visitors, employees, and staff."

Carole uses magic, puppetry, sight gags and much improvisation in her hospital visits at Stevens Hospital (Lynnwood, WA) and the outpatient clinics of Seattle Children's Hospital and Regional Medical Center.

Not everyone can do it

Chris Montross, recreation therapist and a caring clown at St. Luke's Hospital, Cedar Rapids, Iowa, agrees.

"Being a hospital clown is not something that everybody can do," says Chris. "It takes a very special person. The hospital can be a scary place and hospital clowns need to be able to gear themselves to a change of emotions and to gear themselves to the situation at the moment."

Emotional considerations are greater

Emotional considerations of your "audience" are greater. Unlike other types of clowning, sometimes your "audience" is one person. Patients experience greater physical and emotional stress, which affects the way they receive what you offer.

Also, you need to be able to manage your own emotions during difficult situations. "It's important to be able to distance yourself from your feelings at the time in order to assist with the situation," says Louise Weldon, R.N.

Know your limits and trigger points

Every person who clowns has certain triggers and sensitivities to something. It's important to know yourself so you can tap into your real strengths and know which situations you might choose to avoid.

For instance, clowns whose sensitivities may overwhelm them in a pediatric unit or emergency room may wish to clown instead in a transitional care area where patients have less acute conditions. Your clown service can also benefit a hospital in its community relations outreach.

Questions to ask yourself

If you are considering clowning on treatment floors, ask yourself the following questions:

Can I manage my emotions during difficult situations?

Am I comfortable with the medicinal odors often found in hospitals?

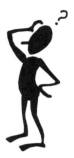

Am I comfortable clowning with people who are in various stages of illness, from mild to critically ill, and with those experiencing various levels of pain?

Am I comfortable with the various noises in a hospital—for instance, the beeping of machines, phones ringing, emergency sirens —and am I able to not be distracted by them?

Will seeing people undergoing various nursing treatments and/or medical procedures be unsettling to me, i.e. people with IV's, nasal tubes, monitors etc.

The bottom line is: Know yourself. Know your hospital.

Understand the Hospital Environment
And Your Place in it

To know if hospital clowning is for you, you need to understand not only yourself and the type of clowning you prefer but also the very special requirements of the hospital environment and how you, as a clown, fit into it.

Learn about the hospital process
"You need to learn what the hospital process is all about," says Suzanne DeTuerk, Director of Volunteer Services at Centre Community Hospital, State College, PA.

"When you think of a clown, you don't think first of a hospital clown but of a circus clown and many people don't know the place that clowns have as part of a patient's care or a family's relief from stress."

A hospital clown needs to understand how people react when they have a loved one in the hospital or are in the hospital themselves for treatment.

It's not like home
"Being in a hospital is not like being at home," Suzanne DeTuerk says. "At home people are surrounded with familiar things –plants, pets, pillows, and family, but in the hospital, people are frightened—they're afraid they will lose their identity and become just a statistic or an ailment. Hospital clowns can allay a patient's fears, especially for younger or elderly patients."

People are vulnerable
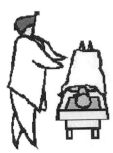
Rev. MaryRuth Smith, a pastoral counselor and former hospital chaplain, notes that with hospital patients, "You have taken their wallet, their jewelry, their professional garb. They are totally disrobed in every spiritual, emotional and physical sense and are extremely vulnerable and ready for someone to bring a covering to them."

Their position is prone

"Their position is prone," says Rev. MaryRuth Smith. "Even if they are in a chair, they are lower than the visitor. But they are the leader and what you respond to is the Spirit of God within their spirit. If you recognize the Spirit in yourself, you'll find it in the patient. The real interaction you have with them is a relationship of Spirit."

Be part of the treatment team

"We want to make people comfortable and at ease," says Suzanne DeTuerk. "They aren't just our 'patients' – they're people."

"The whole idea of hospital clowns is to be part of the treatment team, not just volunteers and not just clowns. They must take their lead from the staff, nurses, doctors, ancillary personnel and the patient, family and friends, in doing all they can to make each person comfortable. Not every clown has to be lighthearted, but you do have to be caring and sensitive to the patient's needs."

Leaders from prominent therapeutic clown programs emphasize how important it is to be part of the hospital wellness team.

Jane "Dr. Tickles" Abendschein, *(right),* Director of the Clown Docs Program at St. Louis Children's Hospital, notes that "one thing that has helped the acceptance of the Clown Docs program at the hospital has been our willingness to become part of the 'wellness team' and to not use humor to undermine the authority of the other staff."

The Clown Docs Program provides a unique opportunity to influence the future of medicine through its work with students at Washington University School of Medicine. First year medical students taking the school's credit selective course on "The Medicine of Laughter" shadow the Clown Docs on their clown rounds to observe the effects of humor in the hospital setting. (for more see p. 71.)

Earn and build trust with the medical staff

"We are considered part of the wellness team and that does not come automatically-- it must be earned," says Aviva "DR Huggabubbe" Gorstein of the Bumper "T" Caring Clowns. She served for 12 years as Director of Volunteer Services for the Vanderbilt Medical Center in Nashville, Tennessee.

Korey Thompson, Artistic Director of Clowns for Children's Hospital of Wisconsin in Milwaukee notes that clowns must build trust with the medical staff.

"There is a mutual respect that grows as staff and clown work together over time," says Korey. "You work through high census days, impromptu birthday parties, and tornado alerts. You meet staff at funerals and at sock hops in the cafeteria."

Understand what a caring clown is and does

So different is a hospital clown from a traditional circus or stage clown that the terms "therapeutic" or "caring" are often used to describe them.

"I feel there is a distinctive difference in the clown as entertainer and one who is working in a healing environment," says Joan "Bunky" Barrington, Coordinator of the Therapeutic Clown Program at The Hospital for Sick Children, who adds "not all clowns working in hospitals are trained specifically or present themselves as specialized 'therapeutic' clowns."

Richard Snowberg describes the caring clown:

"Being a caring clown means that one is caring and a clown. You are not a clown that cares, but rather a caring individual that is a clown. The emphasis and importance is in being caring. It just so happens that your caring persona is as a clown.

"You need to place that caring aspect of your role in first place when entering a room and beginning to interact with a patient/resident. You are there to meet their needs in any way you can. It might be through entertainment. However, it might just be as a compassionate listener. You might not be funny but invaluable at this particular time in someone's life."

Ten Keys to the Caring Clown   Clown Camp® Notebook [6]

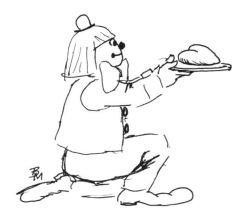

Be a humble servant

Curt "Doctor ICU" Patty of the St. Louis Clown Docs says "You have to be this humble servant. For instance, you might be called to just stand with someone. One time I was in a room where a grandmother was having a difficult time listening to the sounds as the medical staff put an IV line into her granddaughter and I just went and put my arm around her because she couldn't handle the sounds."

Different than a theatre clown

"What makes a hospital clown different from a theatre clown is a sense of service," says Shobhana Schwebke aka "Shobi Dobi," editor of The Hospital Clown Newsletter.

"Hospital clowns give up attachments to results of our performances, as a patient falls asleep in mid show or a doctor walks into a room or any number of interruptions.

"We are there for the patient, not to show off a performance. We often never see the results of our actions until days later, if at all. By the nature of our job, we do not even expect results from our actions. This is selfless service.

"When we say, 'how can I serve you' we offer what we have. It is not about status. It is about compassion. Egos are not involved here."

Chapter 3
Discovering Your Role

Five Roles of a Caring Clown

Stars are lights that shine in the darkness. They don't make the darkness go away but they offer hope and encouragement in the midst of darkness.

They inspire a sense of wonder. They lift our gaze upward. They take us out of ourselves.

As a caring clown, you can bring light into the night. With your smile and caring, you can lighten the spirits of all you meet.

But the true "star" of your clown interaction is the person you clown for, be they patient, family or staff. They are the focus of all you do. They get top billing. In your eyes, they are "the star" on whom your light shines.

The star model

Our visual model of a star presents five key roles of the hospital clown. These are five "touch points" where you as a clown may connect with each person as:

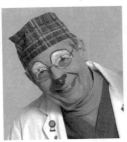

friend
playmate
therapeutic clown
pastoral listener
entertainer

You can combine and blend these roles to meet the unique needs of each person you encounter.

"The star model teaches our students to focus on the various roles of the clown" says Bob "Dr. Bucket" Bleiler (above) of the Bumper "T" Caring Clowns (see p. 60). They use this star model in their classes and mentoring outings to hospitals.

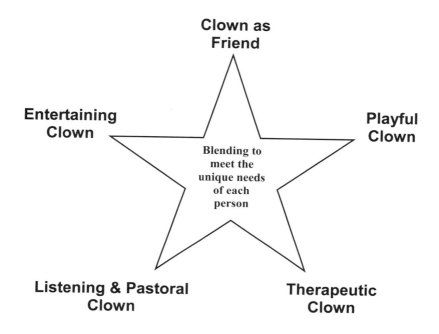

Clown as Friend

Entertaining Clown

Playful Clown

Blending to meet the unique needs of each person

Listening & Pastoral Clown

Therapeutic Clown

No Single Prescription

The star model is not meant to imply a prescription for clowning. With the wide diversity of hospital programs and individual clown skills, there is no single prescription or universal standard for hospital clowning today.

But just as ancient mariners charted their paths by looking at the stars, so we offer this star model to help you chart your own clowning emphasis.

These five ways of being and relating are not exclusive or all encompassing. One often leads to another or blends with another. For instance, listening is therapeutic. Play develops friendship. The different roles can be combined in a galaxy of possibilities.

Each illustrates ways of thinking about how the hospital clown can interact with patients, family and staff. Each also emphasizes certain of the "unspoken messages" present in all caring clown efforts and offers examples of real life experiences.

The Clown as Friend

In attitude and action, the clown as friend is communicating these unspoken messages:
"I like you."
"I want to be your friend."
"I'm here with you."

Be a silent presence

A clown is invited into the room of an elderly woman in her fourth hospitalization. As the clown is asked to her bedside, the woman holds out her hand.

The clown rests her hand under the woman's hand while the woman begins to cry. The clown, in silent presence, is the woman's friend.

(Infection Control Note: This hospital permitted clowns to physically hold a person's hand and then to wash hands afterwards. Be vigilant in following your hospital's infection control rules.)

Show simple caring

"If you say 'hello, I like your outfit, or your shirt,' you show that someone cares about them, that they have a friend," says Curt "Doctor ICU" Patty of the St. Louis Clown Docs.

The clown as friend can reach adults as well as children. Notes Shobhana "Shobi Dobi" Schwebke,

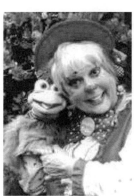

(shown below), editor of *The Hospital Clown Newsletter:*

"Because we are not asking for anything or administering anything, often we step into that warm and fuzzy place of a trusted friend.

"How often after doing a goofy magic trick, an adult will just open up to me and a real bond is made...In the same way children share stories and secrets with my puppets and we all become family."

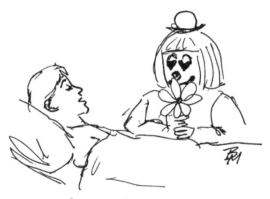

Love with your eyes
Clowns as friends communicate with their eyes.
The clown as friend is willing to step into another's world and enter into another's loneliness.

> *"The clowns are remarkable, not only for their*
> *ability to bring joy, laughter and happiness,*
> *but also for their ability to sit in empathetic silence*
> *with a critically or terminally ill patient,*
> *sharing the comedy and tragedy of humanity*
> *with one another by a tear, a hug, or a gentle touch."*

> —Barbara Anne McCarty, CCLS, Child Life Specialist,
> The Children's Regional Hospital at Cooper Hospital,
> New Jersey speaking of the Bumper "T" Caring Clowns

Make a memory
Just as with any friend, your clown's visit may be remembered long after you leave. As Richard "Snowflake Junior" Snowberg has observed:

> *"Never overlook the significance of your presence to someone you visit.*
> *"Just because you don't know them personally doesn't mean you don't have the same impact as a close personal friend.*
> *"You provide joy and something to talk about after you've gone."*

Crayon drawing (at left) by a 5 year-old after an appearance by "Toot" the clown aka Anita Thies.

The Playful Clown

In attitude and action, the playful clown is communicating these unspoken messages:
"I delight in you."
"I enjoy you."
"I have fun with you."

Every clown offers the opportunity of play, but for some, the majority of their service is that of the playful clown.

The playful clown offers patients a time to reconnect to the fun side of living, if only for moments. This can provide mental and emotional relief and a welcomed escape.

Give a "time out" from pain

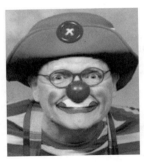

"Your large cartoon-like character can take them out via your fantasy," says Richard "Snowflake Junior" Snowberg *(shown at left)*

"You can remove them from their pain for a time as you playfully involve them in your stories, character and props.

They likely haven't been experiencing any fun. You can fill that need."

Take the inner child "out to play"

Whereas the entertaining clown often carries the whole energy of the relationship themselves, the playful clown invites more interaction. In so doing, the playful clown invites the "inner child" out to play.

"The hospital clown today is the experiential playmate. We give the experience of the moment," says Shobhana Schwebke, aka "Shobi Dobi" the Clown.

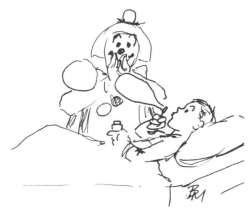

"It is the gift we get and it is our gift to those suffering. It is the gift of play we bring to hospitalized patients and staff and relatives," says Shobi. "Because right then, with you, they can connect to that inner child and to the moment, to that inner glow, that love, that universal connection." [7]

"My kid is back!"

The impact of the playful clown often extends to family members. St. Louis Clown Docs member Curt "Doctor ICU" Patty recalls a time when his wife, Diana "Nurse Sniggles" Patty *(right)* was blowing bubbles for a young girl in intensive care.

At one point the girl reached up and grabbed a bubble and a parent who had been keeping a bedside vigil exclaimed "my kid is back!"

The essence of the playful clown comes from deep within every clown. Once again, "Shobi Dobi" says it best:

Our sense of play makes us fun

"The costume and face may be funny," says Shobi, "but it is our sense of play that makes us fun. We can't afford to lose this play, especially in the hospital where we can't depend on a stage show. It's one-on-one and heart-to-heart. We have to share our own self." [8]

The Therapeutic Clown

In attitude and action, the therapeutic clown is communicating these unspoken messages:
"I support you."
"I encourage you."
"I want to help empower you."

Supporting medical exams

A clown is invited into a treatment room where a 4-year-old girl is being evaluated for a possible concussion. The doctor needs the girl to look up so he can examine the lower part of her eyes with a light. But the girl won't look up. Could the clown help? The clown blows bubbles to the ceiling. The girl follows the bubbles with her eyes and the doctor finishes his exam.

In another instance, a doctor needs to do deep stitches on a teenager's gashed arm. The clown is invited to be a calming presence prior to and after the stitching. The clown does visual magic to divert the teen's attention and afterwards affirms how brave the teen was to tolerate the pain.

A spoonful of clowning helps the medicine go down

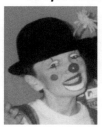

Korey Thompson, *(left)*, Artistic Director of the Clowns for Children's Hospital of Wisconsin, recalls situations when clowns are utilized as potential anti-emetics.

Sometimes patients can be distracted from the upchuck mode at the sight of a clown and at the invitation to play. In one instance, medical staff waited to administer medications that could cause stomach upset until the clown was present. The patient and clown played together for half an hour and the medications didn't inauspiciously reappear.

"For clowns to be used that way, medical staff must have both a trust and understanding of what a clown might potentially offer to the situation," says Korey.

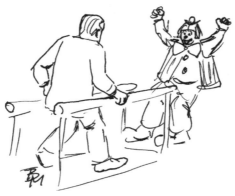

In all of these cases, the hospital clown serves in a therapeutic role to support the medical team in a specific effort. The role of the therapeutic clown is to give a supportive arm and voice to encourage strength and action in others.

While all hospital clowning can be viewed in a broad sense as therapeutic, some hospitals have specialized clown therapists who are Child Life Workers or work with staff as a Clown Therapy Program.

Booking clinics around clown days

One such example is the Therapeutic Clown Program at The Hospital for Sick Children in Toronto, which is under the umbrella of the Child Life Department.

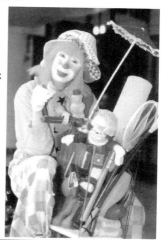

"In our chronic care facility, we often interact with the same patients over a long period of time," says Joan "Bunky" Barrington, *(right)*, Therapeutic Clown Program Coordinator.

"The patients know what days we will be in house (they will book their clinics around clown days) and they trust that we will 'be there' for them. We hold sacred our relationships and their trust in us."

The Listening / Pastoral Clown

In attitude and action, the listening clown is communicating these unspoken messages:
"I hear you."
"I value you."
"I respect you."

"Can you listen to my feelings?"

A clown who is also a trained hospice volunteer stops by the room of an elderly man. His daughter follows the clown into the hallway and says, "they tell us my father will die tonight. I need someone to listen to my feelings right now. Can you?" After clearing it with the nursing staff, the clown leads the woman to a quiet corner to listen.

The clown takes off her clown hat and ping pong ball "nose" and shifts gears into the role of compassionate, reflective listener.

Afterwards the clown gives the woman's daughter some clown stickers and handouts which the woman later says provided relief for her daughter during the roller coaster evening the family experienced. Several days later, the clown—this time in street clothes-- attends the memorial service as a follow up act of caring with the family.

Give an "ear" to another

The role of the listening clown is to literally "give an ear" to receive another's story. The willingness to let someone unburden the heaviness in their heart can be a first step for release.

"I have found many children and adults who are afraid of surgery, patients who were facing serious decisions, patients who were facing the shadow of death," says Desi "Dizzy" Payne, *(left),* who clowns at the Ottumwa (Iowa) Regional Health Center.

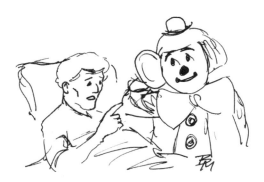

One does not need formal training to be a good listener. Nor do you need to "step out" of clown makeup to listen. Sometimes a family member or patient just wants to talk or share a story with the clown at hand.

Such was the case with a World War II veteran visited by "Americlown," a clown character created by Chris Montross after September 11. Chris, a recreation therapist at St. Luke's Hospital in Cedar Rapids Iowa, recalls:

"I gave this proud veteran a small American flag and he said 'I haven't had a flag of my own for 50 years.'

"He then vented some deep seated memories that weighed heavy on his heart. He allowed himself to cry and helped put some of his feelings into proper perspective.

"A unit nurse later told me that this experience was a dose of much needed medicine for this gentleman."

Make the most of the moment

To listen well, one needs to be open to the moment.

"We don't enter a room with any pre-conceived 'schtick' to do," says Esther "DR Curly Bubbe" Gushner, *(right),* of the Bumper "T" Caring Clowns.

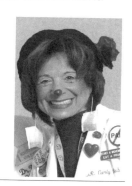

"We know we can't change the diagnosis or the prognosis of the patient. All we have is the moment and in that moment we have the unique opportunity to enhance the hospital environment one person at a time, one smile at a time."

The Entertaining Clown

*In attitude and action, the entertaining clown
is communicating these unspoken messages:*
"I'm here to give to you."
"Escape with me."
"May I entertain you?"

Provide a new focus

A clown is asked to visit a severely injured young man whose father was killed in the same traffic accident that hospitalized him. His mother and sister sit at his bedside. The clown does several brief magic tricks and quietly plays a song on kazoo as requested by his mother. As the clown entertains, the man opens his eyes and smiles for the first time since being hospitalized.

In this instance, the clown carries the entire energy level and focus through entertainment. This is the entertaining clown and there are many ways to be one.

Take them away

With voice, mime or music, the entertaining clown uses all their senses and skills in storytelling, magic, puppets or whatever their specialty to help focus the patient's attention away from their illness and situation.

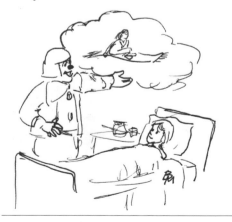

*"In this world of make-believe
Mime and magic, fantasy,
A clown is a friend
you can hold in your heart
A friendship forever
that will never part."*

From the song "Clowns are
God's Children Too"
by Christine Montross

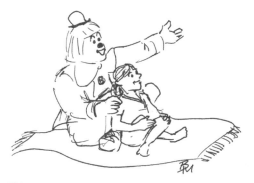

Give them a fantasy experience

As Richard Snowberg notes:

"The word 'entertain' means to focus attention.

"The caring clown is one that helps the audience of one or one hundred focus their attention...

*"Their focusing on your foolishness,
humor and stories
can release them,
even perhaps but for a short time,
from the pain they are suffering.*

*"You are the entertainment.
You are the escape artist,
offering the opportunity to a bed ridden patient
to share in your fantasy experience."* [9]

The smiles evoked by an entertaining clown can lift the entire emotional mood in a room.

As Phyllis Diller quipped, (and as artist Amanda Maser of State College, PA models for us in picture at right):

**A smile is a *curve*
that sets everything straight!**

Chapter 4
Knowledge You Need

Infection control:
First and Always

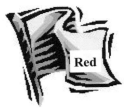

This "red flag" issue is of paramount importance, both for the safety of every person you clown with and for your own health and well-being.

Hospital clowns need to adhere diligently to the same Infection Control Policies and Procedures as their medical team colleagues in specialized environments.

Best practice hospital clowning
must reflect
best practice infection control measures.

One example is the adjustment being made in those hospitals dealing with Severe Acute Respiratory Syndrome (SARS).

"We are formally outlining where we can adjust our practice of therapeutic clowning to comply with the infection control guidelines for SARS," notes Joan "Bunky" Barrington, Coordinator of the Therapeutic Clown Program at The Hospital for Sick Children, Toronto. "We adhere to infection control policies as responsible professionals working with chronic care children."

Illness in a small world

The practice of therapeutic clowning is continuing to evolve. "We are a small world now," notes Joan "and we have to accept what goes with that and adjust. If it's not SARS it may be West Nile Virus or some other illness."

Infection control "at a whole new level"

"Infection control has always been important, but it is practiced at a whole new level now," says Korey Thompson, Artistic Director of Clowns for Children's Hospital of Wisconsin at Milwaukee.

"All indications are that protocols will become more rather than less rigorous for some time to come," Korey says, adding:

"With the number of bad bugs that are resistant to the antibiotics currently available, the need to observe more comprehensive measures is necessary to protect patients, families, staff, AND the clowns. This is not the time or place for casual practice, however well-meaning."

"Learn to love with your eyes and your voice and don't spread disease with your touch." — Janet "Jelly Bean" Tucker

Where to begin

Meet with the person in your hospital who oversees infection control issues. We recommend you:

Review all of your props, costuming and practices with the hospital staff to be sure you are in compliance with every infection control procedure.

You may be surprised at what you learn about the spread and control of germs and illness—airborne and by touch—and how you may need to adapt your clowning and prop use accordingly.

For instance, our local hospital prefers we not blow bubbles by mouth when we are close to patients — so we use manual squeeze devices for bubbles instead.

Ask your hospital about latex issues, feather dusters, clown wigs and how to best transport your props.

Basic Infection Control for Hospital Clowns

Your own hospital is your authority. These are some basic rules at many hospitals:

- Wash hands upon entering and leaving the hospital.
- Don't wear gloves.
- Wash hands after each direct contact with a patient or a patient's belongings. (Some hospitals may prohibit any physical contact for hygiene reasons.)
- Don't re-use anything that falls on the floor.
- Don't put your props on a patient's bed or bed table.
- Give any clown props touched by a patient to that patient to keep or don't use them again until they are disinfected.
- Clean your props and costume after each visit.

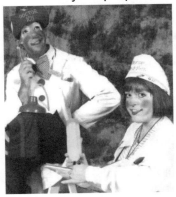

Curt and Diana Patty of the St. Louis Clown Docs *(left)* note that hospital clown props should be made of latex free materials that are easy to cleanse.

"Animal balloons should normally not be taken into the hospital due to the latex allergies of many patients," adds Curt.

Keep educated on issues

An excellent and extensive discussion of hospital infection control and hygiene issues is included in The Hospital Clown: A Closer Look. Current issues also are regularly reported in the Hospital Clown Newsletter. (See page 75.)

Also for your own safety

If your hospital doesn't already require it, be sure to get a TB test, a regular flu shot and any other recommended preventative inoculations.

Patient Privacy and Confidentiality

Hospital clowns worldwide have always emphasized respecting a patient's privacy and confidentiality.

Now within the United States, guarding private health information isn't just an ethical concern; it is a legal one.

HIPAA Patient Privacy Rules

The medical privacy rule of the Health Insurance Portability and Accountability Act (HIPAA) took effect in April, 2003 in the United States. The act mandates a host of regulations protecting patient privacy.

Learn from your hospital staff all the ways that this act impacts on how you relate to patients in your hospital.

The law gives added import to treating as confidential all information which you (or others) may hear directly or indirectly concerning a patient.

Keep it confidential

It means you should never seek information in regard to a patient and never talk about a patient while you are in elevators, hallways or any place for that matter. It means you never reveal a patient's identity.

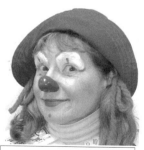

One clown in a small town hospital often encounters patients she knows but while in clown she never acknowledges who she is "as a person" or that she recognizes them. She keeps her knowledge to herself.

"What you see or hear, leave it here"

Betty "Dr. I See You" Hodgson (above) State College, PA

"The key to Caring Clowning is sensitivity."
--Carole "Pookie" Johnson

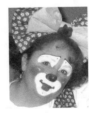

Hospital clowning requires special sensitivity. In fact, sensitivity is at the center of the clown's efforts, much as a clown nose is at the center of a clown's face.

To be sensitive means . . .

To be *sensitive,* says Webster, is to be highly responsive; changing easily or quickly, or delicately aware of the attitudes and feelings of others.

Clowns in hospitals must be sensitive to:

- Health and hygiene concerns
- Hospital rules and constraints
- The needs of patients, family, visitors and staff
- Yourself and what you are comfortable with

Setting guidelines

We invite you to use this chapter as one resource in writing your own hospital clown program guidelines.

Mary "SnickerDoodle" O'Brien, *(left)* Coordinator of the Fun E Bone Repair Unit in Idaho, advises those wanting to start clowning to "find out how other programs are running, nail down the generally accepted standards of practice for hospital clowning, and create a policy and procedure document that describes what you will and will not do at the hospital.

"Make an appointment with the Director of Volunteers (or appropriate person) and let them add their own requirements to it at the very beginning, with the understanding that the document is fluid and will undergo changes as needed. As you establish trust with them, they will be watching your clowning skills, yes; but more so they will be watching to see if you really are concerned about the welfare of their consumers."

20 sensitive issues

Hospital clowns need to be sensitive to:

Basic matters:
- Infection control
- Other health and hygiene issues
- Patient privacy and confidentiality
- Physical touch
- Helping the patient understand your role

Approaching people and situations
- Cultural diversity
- How you approach people
- The adjustment time needed by others
- Social distance space
- Crowding in a room
- Medical procedures

Interacting with patients and others
- The patient's energy levels
  and nonverbal cues
- Each room's situation; each person's needs
- The impact of your clown makeup
- Noise levels
- The length of your visit
- The emotional climate
- The needs of staff
- All hospital rules
- What to say and not say
  ("Foot in mouth" disease)

Be sensitive to patient privacy

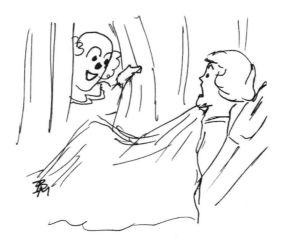

In addition to the patient privacy rules on page 35, be sensitive to the personal feelings of patients.

One thing that people surrender during hospitalization is their privacy. Complete strangers have access to their bodies, and private space and modesty is at a premium.

Please respect closed curtains. Treat every hospital room as an individual's home. [10]

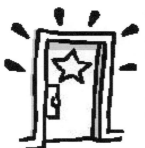

Remember they are "the star"

As we discussed in Chapter 3, please remember that the person you are visiting is the "star" of the interaction.

Thus every room you enter is a "star's" room.

Be sensitive to physical touch

In addition to the infection control and hygiene issues surrounding hand holding and hugs, be insightful about the appropriateness of physical touch.

Help the patient understand your role

Many patients may only have seen clowns in the circus or performing. They may not know what to expect of you and may wonder if you will be loud or intrusive. You need to be sensitive to their concerns and explain who you are and why you are visiting them.

Be sensitive to cultural diversity

"Since September 11, there is a deeper awareness of the need to be sensitive to other cultures and to embrace a multinational understanding," says Korey Thompson, Artistic Director of Clowns for Children's Hospital of Wisconsin in Milwaukee.

"For clowns working in a hospital setting, this means honoring the fact that our experience is only one way of being in the world," says Korey.

"For instance, something we interpret as innocuous such as the hand signal for "A-OK" might have a different meaning in another tradition.

"If there seems to be an unexpected or more-than-average response to a gesture, be alert to the fact that you may be communicating something you don't necessarily intend and tread lightly."

Be sensitive in how you approach people

"I think it is very important for new hospital clowns to learn to have their 'antennae' up at all times," notes Desi "Dizzy" Payne who clowns at the Ottumwa (IA) Regional Medical Center.

"That means to be sensitive to the needs of everyone they come into contact with, whether that is a patient, family member, visitor, or staff member."

Questions You Can Ask Yourself

For example, Desi says, before you approach patients, ask yourself:

- Do they seem afraid of clowns?

- Are they sick to their stomach or in pain and would not like a visit at this time?

- Are they inviting you in by their facial expressions?

- Is there happiness or grief in the room?

- Did they just receive bad news?

Ways to announce your arrival

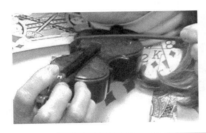

One way is to play soft music. Betty "Dr. I See You" Hodgson plays a "magic strings violin" outside the room and at the door to announce her presence before patients see her.

Do not startle or surprise!

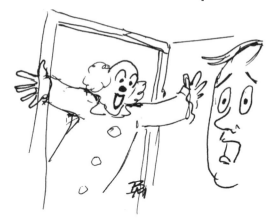

More correct ways to announce your arrival

- Play visual hide and seek or peek a boo
- Quietly knock on doors, walls or windows
- Use words
- Approach slowly, make eye contact!
- Invite interactions but don't intrude
- Bridge the distance between you and another with mime, a wave, bubbles, puppets, quiet music
- Wait for an invitation or permission to enter

Be sensitive to the adjustment time needed by others

Give folks a chance to size you up.

Look around their room or comment on something in their room as a springboard for conversation. In doing so, you give the patient time to evaluate you.

Remember, they weren't expecting you and may be quite taken aback.

Be sensitive to social distance space

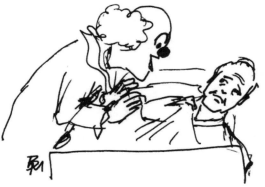

Once you have been invited into a room, allow the patients their "space." (They can't back up or move very far!) Do your clowning from a respectful distance.

"*It's essential for clowns visiting a hospital to learn to feel when they are or are not invading another's space,*" says Janet "Jelly Bean" Tucker who has written:

When a child panics . . .
"*The child who laughs at the clown at 8 feet away but screams and panics when the clown approaches 3 feet is reacting to space invasion.*

. . .retreat to a safe distance
"*The message for the clown in this case is retreat, usually as rapidly as possible, then from a "safe" distance do a trick and wait for acceptance by the child and an invitation to come closer.*

. . .and wait for a new invitation
"*When you feel another person draw back or turn away, stop and retreat back one step. In a few moments you may feel invited to step closer but always wait for the invitation.*" [11]

Social distance increases

You should have developed sensitivity about social distance BEFORE beginning hospital clowning. Unlike children playing outdoors, hospitalized patients cannot get away from you if you invade their space.

Social distance space increases more in a hospital because of the physical and emotional needs of the patients.

Be sensitive to crowding in a room

Don't crowd people in a room for more reasons than one! Also be aware of the placement of medical machines.

Be sensitive to medical procedures

Ask permission if a medical person enters - they may want you to leave while they are adjusting machines etc. If a patient is in need of assistance, notify the nurse's station (do not aid them yourself).

Be sensitive to the patient's energy levels and non-verbal cues

The least energy required of the patient may be to have the patient listen to you with their eyes closed or simply to watch you.

Don't assume, if you're being ignored, that they want to ignore you. They may not have the strength to visit with you at the time. Allow them to make the choice.

People in pain or discomfort, tired or extremely weak, may not desire long conversation. The best visits reflect sensitivity to a patient's state of mind, to drooping eyes or restlessness. Arranging to return at another time is one solution. Sleeping patients should always be allowed to rest.[12]

Be sensitive to each room's situation and the needs of each person

"Read" the room. Every room may require a different approach. Assess each situation and its possibilities.

As a hospital clown, you can "play" off the environment. Many clowns learn storytelling and improvisation. Others share a laugh, a little magic, a joke or a smile.

Don't overlook just talking. Learn to just listen if that is what is needed. Try and leave a memory (photo, sticker, coloring page, a prescription for hugs). Expect the unexpected.

"In a caring clown situation, you have an audience of from one to four persons," says Richard "Snowflake" Snowberg. *"You attempt to meet their needs with an escape from boredom or pain, compassion, a listening ear or whatever is needed by this one person. These are strategies which you'd never consider when doing a company picnic."*

Be sensitive to the impact of your makeup

Some clown faces were meant for long distance stage work, not close up visits. Some hospital clowns wear partial makeup without wigs. Your makeup and costume should not be scary.

Remember that some adults are traumatized for life because they were scared by clowns as a child! For more on clown makeup in hospitals, see Chapter 5.

Be sensitive to noise levels

The hospital clown is quieter. Loud or startling noises are inappropriate.

Be sensitive to the length of your visit

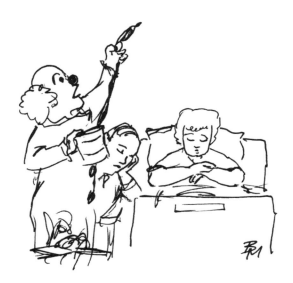

- Don't overstay or drain their energy.
- Be aware of time. (Up to 10 minutes per patient)
- Know when the show "shouldn't go on."

 ## Be sensitive to the emotional climate in hallways, elevators and waiting rooms

One family may be in joy; another family in grief. Also pay attention to family, friends and healthcare providers. They need you too!

 ## Be sensitive to the needs of staff

"Originally hospitals brought us in to entertain the patients," notes Joe "Doc Geezer" Barney, "but I find we tend to have as much impact on the staff as the patients."

Avoid "foot in mouth" disease
(what not to say)

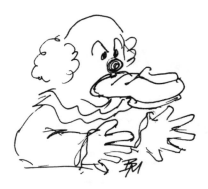

- ❖ Do not ask how patients are unless you are well prepared for the answer.
- ❖ Do not sit or lean on their bed, and do not touch any equipment.
- ❖ Avoid shallow talk. ("I know just how you feel")
- ❖ Avoid insincere promises. ("You'll be better by tomorrow")

Be sensitive to <u>all</u> hospital rules

Reach your hospital contact person and make arrangements to meet with them and their infection control specialist.

Research how you can become part of their healing wellness team.

Ways to grow in sensitivity

- Clown with a partner (4 eyes in a room are better than 2).
- Take "listening" training through hospice or pastoral care.
- Take improvisational training to be more aware of your surroundings and environment.

Chapter 5
Clown Makeup and Costuming

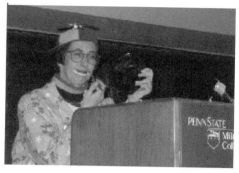

Anita "Dr. Duck" Thies demonstrates minimal clown makeup during an educational presentation to The Healing Arts Student Interest Group at the Penn State College of Medicine, Hershey, PA *Michelle Tillander photo, used with permission*

Makeup: a little goes a long way

Currently, there are no uniform standards for hospital clowns in either makeup or costuming. There are, however, makeup guidelines that distinguish hospital clowns from more traditional circus and theatre clowns.

The faces of circus and theatre clowns were designed to be seen at a distance. Their makeup often is too bold for close up work in hospitals. The hospital clown needs a gentler face to bring joy and caring to vulnerable patients.

In recent years, many clowns have redesigned their faces for hospital work to feature more minimal makeup. "We wear just enough makeup so that the patients realize we're not real doctors but fun doctors," says DR Bumper "T" *(below).*

"Our makeup is very, very soft makeup. It is less than what is known as the 'European clown face,'" he says. "We look just other-worldly enough so that patients immediately feel comfortable sharing their feelings and concerns with us."

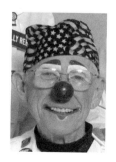

"The only thing all of our Bumper "T" Caring Clowns have in common with our clown cousins is our red nose." —DR Bumper "T"

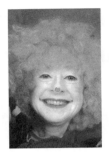

A gentle "whiteface" look

Some hospital clowns are "whiteface" clowns with a very gentle look.

An excellent example is Camilla "Posy" Gryski, *(left),* a therapeutic clown at The Hospital for Sick Children in Toronto.

As you design your clown face

Your hospital clown face should bring out your special sparkle, your whimsical look, your winsome smile.

Your makeup should reveal, not cover up. Spend time looking in a mirror to see how your own face muscles work. Then place makeup where it will emphasize and move with your natural expressions.

Markings at the laugh lines near your mouth or eyes may be enough. You may need very little white. See how little makeup you can apply for maximum effect.

When looking at clown makeup resources, remember that many are targeted for traditional whiteface, auguste or tramp clowns who serve different audiences.

Learn how to apply makeup correctly and design your face to uniquely meet the needs of your hospital audience.

Notice how an excellent clown face such as that of Peggy "Sunflower" Cole emphasizes expressions and "moves" as she raises her eyebrows (center) or deepens her smile (right).

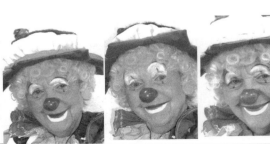

Costumes and characters

Many clowns develop clown "doctor" or "nurse" personas. Many others have clown characters not built on any medical theme. See what works for you and what is best received at your hospital.

Some clown "doctors" use clown names that begin with "doctor" spelled out or "DR" without the period or "Dr." in quotation marks to clearly distinguish themselves from and to not offend "real" medical doctors.

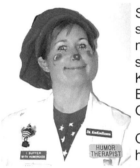

Some clown "doctors" don lab coats and scrubs as part of their outfit, adding to it a number of humorous buttons such as shown by Susie "Dr. KooKooHeimer" Kleinwachter *(left)* or Esther "DR Curly Bubbe" Gushner *(right)*.

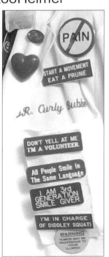

Other clowns enter the hospital as their regular clown or as another character unrelated to medicine. Some clowns believe there is a need for a "counterpoint" to the white coats already walking the hospital corridors.

Be sure it's easy to clean

Whatever your character, your costume should be easily cleanable.

Curt and Diana Patty of the St. Louis Clown Docs note that since a hospital clown's costume will be washed after each day, "it is important that it be easy to take care of. Avoid dresses with fancy slips that could easily get caught in the hospital equipment. Wigs are normally not worn because of the added care necessary to take care of them."

More pictures of clowns are in Chapter 7, page 59.

Chapter 6
Creative Ideas

Developing the Art of Hospital Clowning

The art of the hospital clown is finding your balance. The balance between inner and outer. What you bring inside of you to offer and what the outer situation requires.

It is not something that can be learned solely in the mind. It comes with experience, like riding a bicycle.

It's okay to have training wheels as you learn to find your inner balance. Those training wheels are the steps you can take to practice sensitivity and to practice creativity.

You'll have that inner sense of when you are being sensitive and when you are being creative and when you need to make adjustments to keep the balance.

Remembering the goal of your creativity: Meeting patient needs

The goal of whatever you create as a hospital clown is to meet the individual needs of the patient.

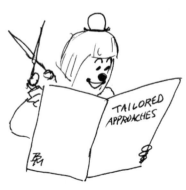

We encourage you to have a vision of that creative process.

Consider these images.

The clown is like an original costumer who "sizes up" each individual and tailors materials to fit what is needed.

The hospital clown is like a dancer who sees someone across the room. The clown assesses the situation and invites permission to approach. The clown approaches, engages, departs.

Let the patient lead

During their time together, the clown lets the patient "lead." Perhaps the clown dances alone or with a clown partner, improvising steps to suit the tone of the room. Perhaps hands lightly touch. Perhaps the patient makes the music.

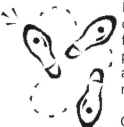

Perhaps the clown dances the "cha-cha" with one foot forward and the other back. Forward for entertainment, back to listen; forward for play, back for friendship. The clown moves according to the patient's needs, taking care not to step on sensitive toes.

Or consider the clown as a chef who first assesses the patient's "dietary" preferences. Low-energy? A need for some sweetness? Something easy to digest?

The clown chef may have brought many ingredients—a smorgasbord of skills—to draw from. But the intent is not to deliver a pre-packaged meal.

Instead, the clown whips up a unique creation from scratch, flavoring it to the taste of the patient.

As you practice the principle "Be Creative"
think how Webster defines "create" as:

* To bring into being from nothing
* To bring about
* To invest with a new function

Growing in Creativity

Develop your clown character

The first gift you bring to hospital patients is the gift of yourself. Begin, then, by expressing yourself through a clown character. There are many resources and workshops that will help you discover the clown in you.

"My suggestion for new clowns is to put all the energy you can into developing your clown character first and then start adding skills," says Mary "SnickerDoodle" O'Brien. "If your clown has no character, even as a beginner, you are just going to be someone dressed up like a clown."

Learn what makes something funny

Study and practice different kinds of humor:
Visual
Spoken
Auditory including musical
Silent
We offer some examples, especially of visual humor, in this chapter. Use them to create your own humor.

Observe what prompts laughter:

❖ Exaggeration
❖ Pushing the extremes of possibility—
   extending something to its illogical conclusion
❖ Incongruity
❖ Failure and overcoming failure with surprising success
❖ Contradiction of the expected
❖ Misuse of words (puns are great!)
❖ Absurdity
❖ Parody of the human situation
❖ Sounds

"A laugh is the shortest distance between two people." Victor Borge

Ideas for visits

How you say it makes it funny

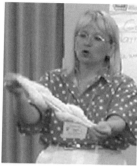

It's **how** you do it, how you say it that often makes it funny.

Consider the laughs that the words "cluck cluck" bring in making the towel chicken as demonstrated by Tammy "Hugz" Miller at left.

"Making the towel chicken works very well with women patients who like to cook," adds Betty "Dr. I See You" Hodgson. "We say we're going to make a chicken but we need the cluck cluck. Just saying "cluck cluck"—that's a funny line."

How to Make the Towel Chicken

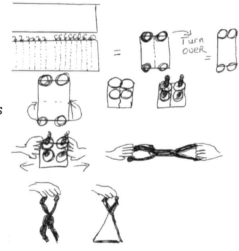

1. Open towel fully

2. Roll each "end" (narrow side--the ends of the rectangle) in to the middle

3. Turn over and fold back in half

4. Pull 4 "end" corners of towel out a little

5. Grasp the 2 "left-side" outside "ends" with fingers on your left hand and the 2 "right side" outside ends with fingers of your right hand and pull

6. Hold up end of "chicken" with one hand. For "dressed" chicken, shake out bottom ends to look like dress.

Ideas for visits

Think visually. Think corny. Think fun. Think of puns. Let these props used by Clowns Doing Rounds stimulate your creative mind.

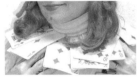
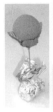

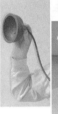
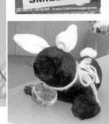

Can you identify. . .

- The stool sample ("take it to pathology," one doctor quipped)
- The diamond necklace (draws quips that "you're not playing with a full deck")
- The nose rose given to patients (uses clown nose)
- The one who is here for a "chick-up"
- The one who came for a "hop-eration" so he wouldn't croak
- The stethoscope
- The variation on a popular pain medicine whose box holds instead strips of jokes to give out
- For older audiences, the Easter seal (with a variation for the Christmas seal)
- "Tickets" given especially to long-term patients and those waiting for tests.

Ticket

___ Operating a wheelchair without a license
___ Operating a hospital bed without training
___ Speeding
___ Eating too much jello
___ Laughing in the hospital
___ Parking (been here too long)

Tell a Good Story

Storytelling, with or without props, is a great way to help patients find new focus. Storyteller Susie Kleinwachter offers these tips.

"Try to make sure you have no interruptions if possible or your story will loose its impact.

"If an interruption does occur, start the story over. Several repetitions of this are really funny.

"Have the story be short and sweet. Happy endings are ALWAYS the best. Keep your voice at a lower tone and encourage patient participation if possible."

Ideas for visits

Here are a few ideas to spark your own:

- Wave, play peek a boo

- Use bubble blow

- Kazoo softly

- Talk to your puppet

- Walk an invisible dog on a leash

- Use simple pocket magic— a thumb tip and disappearing scarf or the magic coloring book

- Use juggling scarves

- Tell puns and corny jokes if the occasion permits

- Take pretend pictures and give away smiley stickers

- Give an "IYQ" eye test with the "secret clown message" which is "I like you" and then give IYQ stickers

- Sing silly songs

- Do visual gags with the rubber chicken including with dice (diced chicken); with a blue cloth and cord (chicken cordon bleu) and with a king's crown (chicken ala king).

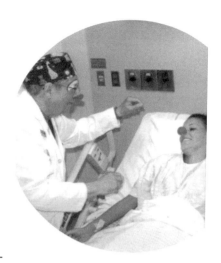

Bob "DR Bucket" Bleiler of the Bumper "T" Caring Clowns performs a "red nose" transplant on a willing volunteer. (Picture used with permission.)

Doing a "red nose" transplant

You can pretend to measure the nose with a "level" to see that the person is "on the level" and to test eye-nose coordination by asking the person to catch a bubble on their nose.

After they have put the nose on, you can pretend to take their picture and give them a smiley sticker with the red nose on it. If you do several transplants at once you can comment on the family "resemblance."

Clown Humor Carts

Rx Laughter Caring Clown Unit
Rochester, New York

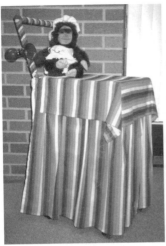

The Rx Laughter Caring Clown Unit of Rochester (NY) General Hospital uses this humor cart to wheel their props around.

Coordinator Debbie Nupp says, "Its main body is a Gracious Living six drawer rolling storage unit. We have added a few features.

"The handle (covered with multi color tape) of the cart came from a stroller and is attached to either side of the cart. We replaced the original wheels of the unit with the dual axle stroller wheels. This made it easier to get in and out of the elevators and much smoother pushing.

"I designed a colorful skirt that resembles a circus tent. It is attached with double sided velcro for easier cleaning. We also have attached a horn. A laundry bag hangs from the side to put props in that might be touched by patients. *(continued)*

Sized for 2 Clowns

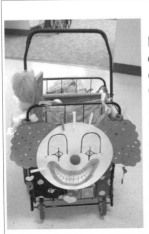

Here is an example of a smaller clown cart used by the Clowns Doing Rounds in State College, PA.

The clowns always clown in teams of two and find this size just right for their needs.

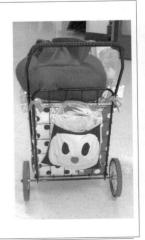

Perfect height for bedridden patients

"Added to the front are large hooks screwed into the cart that carry some of the larger props such as the rubber chicken. This cart is small enough to fit in semi-private rooms easily. It is of perfect height for bedridden patients to view magic tricks which are done on top of the cart."

Props in the cart by drawer:

1. Our humorous prescription cards, my business cards, notebook that contains sample isolation signs, very basic sign language for clowns, and directions for magic tricks. Adhesive tapes to make huggie pillows.

2. This is our sticker drawer designed with dowels to hold the stickers on rolls. This keeps the drawer neat and accessible.

3. This drawer divided in quarters holds our nose transplant items.

4. 5. and 6. These contain our magic tricks, donations from local merchants for give aways to patients and also can be utilized for the clowns to carry around some of their favorite items while on rounds.

A great give away: the napkin rose

Tell a story involving roses as you make this napkin rose to leave with a patient. Quip that it doesn't need water or it's only a paper rose. Or hum "everything's coming up roses' or "tip toe through the tulips" (there's clown humor in being confused). Our thanks to ShaSha the Clown (Sharon Di Tirro) who teaches a variation of this rose using florist tape and based on a free guide posted on the internet.

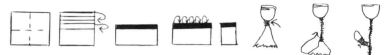

Fully open up napkin; Refold one-half of the napkin by folding down strips of 1 1/2 inches (about 4 strips) until you go just over the center fold of the napkin. Roll the napkin sideways from one side to the other around two fingers starting at the thickened strip area.

Twist under the wrapped part to begin the stem. Twist stem until half way down. Find the loose bottom outside corner and flip it up to simulate a "leaf." Continue twisting beneath "leaf" to finish stem.

Ways to Exit the Room

Look for the positive and leave them with a smile

The Bumper "T" Caring Clowns have a standard way of leaving each patient's room.

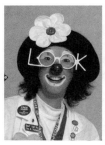

What we do, says Reba "DR Silly Reba" Strong, *(left)*, is say, "It was wonderful visiting with you and before I leave I'd like to tell you that you have three things going for you."

They are:

Number One: "You name something positive you have noticed in the room--be it a pretty blanket, flowers, cards or photographs or a member of the family who is visiting.

"You look for something positive and personal to the patient. If there isn't anything obvious, then you say 'you've got a great smile.'

Number Two: You then say 'you're in a very good hospital' and finally,

Number Three: You say 'I'm not your doctor.' That always gets a laugh."

When checking in and out of the hospital:

1 Upon your arrival at the hospital, check in with the desk and nurses station.
2 Find out if there is anything you need to know.
3 Determine and get approval for appropriate give-aways.
4 Inform the nurses' station when you are leaving and ask if there is anything else you can do.

Chapter 7
Hospital Clowns and Programs

Today, you can learn hospital clowning from many excellent teachers and practitioners. Some programs offer "mentoring" where students "shadow" experienced clowns on their hospital rounds. Major conferences teach best practices in hospital clowning. Many teachers travel nationwide.

This chapter introduces you to some hospital clowns we know who are willing to share their time and expertise with you. This is not an all-inclusive list but represents clowns from throughout the United States and Canada who we believe are setting the standards in hospital clowning. We invite you to contact them.

To learn about more hospital clown programs, see *The Hospital Clown Newsletter* by "Shobi Dobi" and *The Hospital Clown: A Closer Look,* by Shobi and Patty Wooten. (see p. 75)

The Clowns Pictured on the Back Cover (from left in each row)

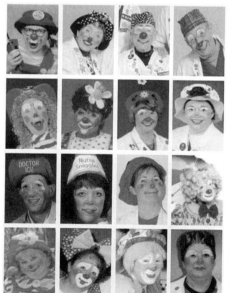

Richard "Snowflake" Snowberg p. 67
Aviva "DR HuggaBubbe" Gorstein p. 60
DR Bumper "T" p. 60
Bob "DR Bucket" Bleiler p. 60

Desi "Dizzy" Payne p. 65
Carole "Pookie" Johnson p. 64
Cathie "DR Periwinkle" Degen p. 60
Denise "DR Dazzles" Black p. 60

Curt "Doctor ICU" Patty p. 68
Diana "Nurse Sniggles" Patty p. 68
Sue "Dr.KooKooHeimer"
      Kleinwachter p. 64
Debbie "Cheerios" Nupp p. 66

Shobhana "Shobi Dobi" Schwebke p. 67
Mary "SnickerDoodle" O'Brien p. 63
Joan "Bunky" Barrington p. 69
Jane "Dr. Tickles" Abendschein p. 68

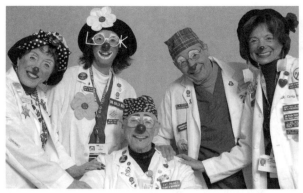

Leaders of The Bumper 'T' Caring Clowns are, from left Aviva "DR HuggaBubbe" Gorstein, Reba "DR Silly Reba" Strong, "DR Bumper 'T' " (seated); Bob "DR Bucket" Bleiler and Esther "DR CurlyBubbe" Gushner (*Alex Linton photo antonimages@aol.com*)

The Bumper "T" Caring Clowns (NJ & PA)

The Bumper "T" Caring Clowns, a 501c3 nonprofit organization headquartered in Barrington, New Jersey, near Philadelphia, trained 50 hospital clowns last year for 10 hospitals in Pennsylvania and New Jersey.

They currently are working with the Association for Applied and Therapeutic Humor and others to raise the bar on acceptable standards for hospital clowns and to develop a national certification procedure for hospital caring clowns.

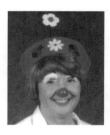

Bumper "T" Clown Cathie "DR Periwinkle" Degen clowns at Bryn Mawr (PA) Hospital

Shadowing is important

"Shadowing is a very important part of our training program," says "DR Bumper 'T'."

"It takes a special approach to work in a hospital and to truly understand how to zero in on a patient's spirit and not be overwhelmed by the sights, sounds and smells of the hospital environment.

"We make the most of the moment one smile at a time. This is something that cannot be learned through a lecture or by reading a book but by experiencing it."

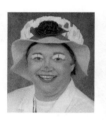

Bumper "T" Clown Denise "DR Dazzles" Black clowns at Paoli (PA) Memorial Hospital

The Bumper "T" Caring Clowns PO Box 37, Barrington, NJ 08007
1-800-280-9544 Email: Caringclowns @tbtcc.org

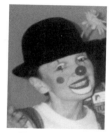

Korey "Tunkal"
Thompson

Clowns for Children's Hospital of Wisconsin

Korey "Tunkal" Thompson
Artistic Director of Clowns
Children's Hospital of Wisconsin in Milwaukee
% 3324 N. Shepard Ave.   Milwaukee, WI 53211
(414) 332-6590   ThompKM@aol.com

Clown Connection (Cedar Rapids, Iowa)

Resource People at St. Luke's Hospital
Chris Montross & Kay Mineck
Pastoral Care Department   St. Luke's Hospital
1026 A. Avenue N.E. Cedar Rapids, Iowa 52402
(319) 369-8082   Chris's email: americlown@mcleodusa.net

Clowns Doing Rounds (State College, PA)

Specially trained hospital clowns from The Happy Valley Alley of the World Clown Association regularly visit Centre Community Hospital in State College, PA in a program the Alley organized called "Clowns Doing Rounds."

Program Director is Betty "Dr. I See You" Hodgson, the Alley's "Vice President of Medicinal Giggles."

The hospital clowns work through the office of the Hospital Volunteer Coordinator. Specialized hospital clown training is required including shadowing. (Three of the hospital clowns have trained at Clown Camp ® University of Wisconsin, La Crosse.)

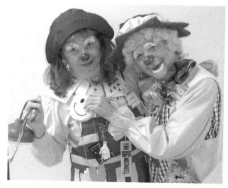

Peggy "Sunflower" Cole (right) uses her smiley stethoscope to check Betty "Dr. I See You" Hodgson

Betty "Dr. I See You" Hodgson
449 Sinking Creek Rd.
Spring Mills, PA 16875
(814) 422-8780
hxz@psu.edu

Clowns on Rounds, Inc. (Albany, NY)

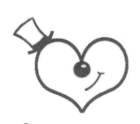

©Clowns on Rounds, Inc.

Clowns on Rounds, Inc.
PO Box 6364
Albany, NY 12206
(518) 861-0128
Email:
eperson@capital.net
Web Site: http://
www.clownsonrounds.com

Clowns on Rounds, Inc. provides professional entertainers dressed as clown doctors and nurses to hospitals and nursing homes in New York State's Capital District.

Funding for this not for profit corporation comes from charitable foundations, corporations and private donations.

The purpose of Clowns on Rounds is:

"to encourage in hospitalized patients, a positive attitude toward their illness and through humor, to help alleviate the fears, anxieties and stress experienced by patients, their families, friends and caregivers."

Executive Director is Elaine Person. Program Director is Loretta DeAngelus.

Loretta DeAngelus aka "Dr. Gigglebritches"

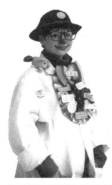

Loretta DeAngelus
"Dr. Gigglebritches"
1063 Valerie Drive
Niskayuna, NY
12309
(518) 272-9197
Email:
DrGbrtchs1@aol.com

Loretta DeAngelus has been a professional and volunteer clown for over 20 years. Loretta's nursing background and her awareness that laughter is the best medicine gave rise to "Dr. Gigglebritches" 10 years ago.

She currently works two days a week as Dr. Gigglebritches at Ellis Hospital and Sunnyview Rehabilitation Center in Schenectady, New York.

Recently, she began a special pilot program for the children in the Albany Medical Center Pediatric Oncology Clinic.

She has been program director for Clowns on Rounds, Inc. since 1998. In 2000, she was named Clown of the Year by Clowns of America International.

In March 2003, she received the "State of New York Women Pioneering the Future Award."

Comedy Connection (Clearwater, Florida)

The Comedy Connection started providing Caring Clowns & Comedy Carts for patients, families and staff in 1988.

Morton Plant Mease Healthcare are JCAHO accredited hospitals (Joint Commission on Accreditation of Healthcare Organizations). They have over 100 hospital volunteers and the clowns are required to take a 10 week training program prior to making rounds.

The Comedy Carts are in operation from noon to 4 p.m. on weekdays and visitors are welcome to join on rounds!

The Comedy Connection is always open for visitors or tours with volunteers.

> The Comedy Connection
> Morton Plant Hospital
> 300 Pinellas St.
> Clearwater, FL 33757
> (727) 462-7841

The Fun E Bone Repair Unit (Boise, Idaho)

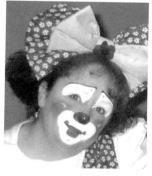

"The Fun E Bone Repair Unit trains, supports, and empowers clowns to serve in various health care related settings," says Coordinator Mary "SnickerDoodle" O'Brien.

As of 2003, 136 people had gone through the unit's annual training program.

"Whether clowning for hospital or hospice patients, seniors, children with special needs, families or staff, Fun E Bone clowns adhere to established 'best practice' guidelines to provide the most ethical and compassionate clowning possible."

Successful weekly programs are in place at Saint Alphonsus Regional Medical Center in Boise; St. Luke's Regional Medical Center in Boise and Meridian, and Mountain States Tumor Institute in Boise.

Giveaways and stickers are provided by grants written to auxiliary organizations. A new weekend program, "Fun E.U." will cover highpoints of their 30-hour training.

> Mary "SnickerDoodle" O'Brien, Coordinator, Fun E Bone Repair Unit
> 3873 South Gideon Place
> Meridian Idaho 83642
> (208) 884-0682
> Email: snicker_d00dle@ mindspring.com
> Note: the 0's are zeroes

"I encourage new clowns to find a mentor—someone who has clowned successfully for a number of years," says Mary. "My first two mentors were online, and I wouldn't have had the courage to follow my dream if Shobi Dobi and Beatrice Buttons hadn't been there with support, ideas and encouragement."

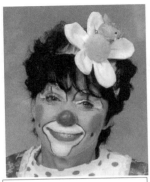

Carole Johnson aka "Pookie"

Carole "Pookie" Johnson is a nationally known Caring Clown and Instructor.

She clowns at nursing homes and at Stevens Hospital (Lynnwood, WA), and makes weekly rounds of the outpatient clinics of Seattle Children's Hospital and Regional Medical Center.

She has been appearing as "Pookie" since 1990. She also specializes in clowning for preschool audiences and for the elderly.

She is a sought after teacher at national conferences who teaches Introduction to Caring Clowning, Props and Routines for Caring Clowns, and Developing the Caring Clown. She also offers one-day Caring Clown Intensives.

Carole Johnson
1602 Locust Way
Lynnwood WA
98036-9017
(425) 481-7143 Email:
clownjuglr@aol.com

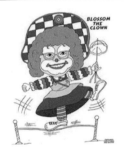

Carole Kay aka "Blossom"

This active Canadian clown has performed extensively. Contact: Carole Kay Box 363 Bradford, Ontario Canada L3Z 2A9   (905) 775-0088 Email: blossomb-b-@on.aibn.com Website: http://www.clownb-b.to/

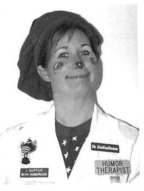

Susie Kleinwachter aka "Dr. KooKooHeimer"

Also known as "Pancakes," this award winning clown, storyteller, and public speaker has taught throughout the US, UK and Canada and recently led a "Health and Humor" workshop in Monterrey, Mexico entitled "Projecto Risa." She is current Membership Director of AATH (Association for Applied and Therapeutic Humor). She sells many items for hospital/nursing home clowning. See p. 80.

Susie "Pancakes" Kleinwachter   PO Box 700 Warrenville, IL 60555 (630) 393-7714 Email: FunE98@aol.com   Website: KleinTime.com

Kettering Medical Center Network (Ohio)
"Anything But Serious" Hospital Clown Troupe

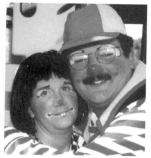

Valerie "Pennies" Haley and
James "Spots" Haley

Valerie Haley
2110 Leiter Rd.
Miamisburg, OH 45342
(937) 384-4884
Email: Valerie.Haley@
kmcnetwork.org

This volunteer clown troupe was the brainchild of Valerie Parker-Haley, an employee of the Kettering Medical Center.

The group originated in the winter of 1999 and currently has more than 45 active clowns. Their mission is to bring encouragement, smiles, and a little bit of cheer to those who need it most.

The clowns all are required to go through the hospital's volunteer department and to attend monthly meetings and ongoing training.

This award-winning troupe is supported by the Kettering Medical Center Network but also accepts donations to help offset supply costs.

The clowns visit nursing homes, hospice, local charities, as well as area hospitals.

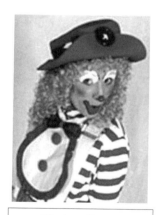

Desirae Payne
2616 Clearview St.
Ottumwa IA 52501
Email: Balloonfactory
@rew2000.com

Ottumwa Regional
Health Center (Iowa)
Desi Payne aka "Dizzy"

Desi Payne, a professional clown since 1995, has been involved with drama and clowning for more than 20 years. She also has worked as a children's pastor.

As "Dizzy the Clown," she brings "Merry Heart Medicine" every week to the Ottumwa Regional Health Center. (ORCH) She is sponsored by the Ottumwa Regional Health Foundation.

Her humor therapy includes singing, telling stories, blowing bubbles, juggling, and using puppets. Her clown mentor, Chuck Rinkel, pioneered clown/humor therapy at ORCH in 1991 as "Dr. Bugg."

Therapeutic Humor Program
Rochester General Hospital
(New York)

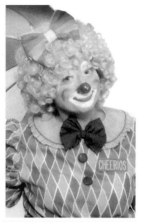

Debbie Nupp
Coordinator
Therapeutic Humor
Program
Rochester General
Hospital
1425 Portland Avenue
Rochester, NY 14621
(585) 922-3596
Email: deb.nupp@
viahealth.org

Coming Soon:
Debbie plans to publish
how to make towels in a
patient's room into dogs,
swans, and more that you
leave with the patient.

Debbie Nupp, LPN, has been a nurse for 25 years, most recently working in the operating room and pediatric unit.

After attending an AATH conference (Association for Applied and Therapeutic Humor), she was inspired to create a humor program in her own hospital, Rochester General Hospital in Rochester, NY.

Launched in 1999 with funding from the Rochester General Hospital Foundation, today the award winning therapeutic humor program has four components:

- Clown Rounds by the Rx Laughter Caring Clown Unit. Since 1999, 31 volunteer clowns have been specially trained for clown rounds.
- A Humor TV channel that shows classic comedies on the hospital closed circuit television 24 hours a day.
- A Humor Library
- Humor Education. "Clownology" courses for new clowns are offered through the year as are classes for staff on the value of humor.

Last year, the Rx Laughter Caring Clown Unit won the New York State Volunteer Award. At the hospital, Debbie works as both a nurse and as coordinator of the therapeutic humor program. She clowns as "Cheerios" the clown.

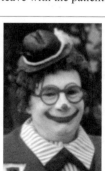

Bud Salloum
aka "Buddy the Clown"
Co-Founder
Edmonton, Canada Caring Clowns
12407-135 Street Edmonton
Alberta, Canada T5L IX8
(780) 455-6049

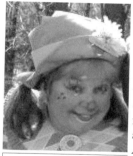

Shobhana Schwebke aka "Shobi Dobi"

Shobhana Schebke, M.A., aka "Shobi Dobi," is a world renowned caring clown, author, teacher, and artist. She is the editor and publisher of *The Hospital Clown Newsletter*, an international newsletter published since 1995. She is the co-author, with Patty Wooten, of *The Hospital Clown: A Closer Look*. (see page 75).

Shobi has worked as a hospital clown at Kaiser Permenante in Oakland, California and in hospitals, clinics and orphanages in Guatemala, India, China and Russia.

She leads hospital clown workshops internationally and also gives laughter workshops.

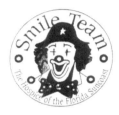

Shobhana Schwebke
aka Shobi Dobi
P.O. Box 8957
Emeryville, CA
94662
(510) 420-1511
Shobidobi@aol.com

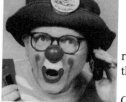

The Smile Team of Hospice of the Florida Suncoast

Joye "TING" Swisher,
300 East Bay Drive Largo, FL 33774
Joyeswisher@thehospice.org,
(727) 586-4432

Dr. Richard Snowberg aka "Snowflake Junior"

Dr. Richard Snowberg is an internationally renowned clown and educator who was inducted into the International Clown Hall of Fame in 1999.

For the past 23 years, he has directed Clown Camp® which he founded at the University of Wisconsin, LaCrosse. An emeriti faculty member at the University of Wisconsin, LaCrosse, he has written five books on clowning including the classic *Caring Clowns: How Humor, Smiles and Laughter Overcome Pain, Suffering and Loneliness* (see p. 75).

He has twice served as President of the World Clown Association, most recently in 2002. He teaches, clowns and travels throughout the world.

Dr. Richard
Snowberg
snowberg.rich@
uwlax.edu
(608) 785-8053
http://
perth.uwlax.edu/

Clown Docs of St. Louis Children's Hospital

Jane Abendschein started the Clown Docs program at St. Louis Children's Hospital in 1999. She is the director for the program that supplies clowns in the clinics and at bedsides. Her Clown Doc name is Dr. Tickles.

Other regular members of the Clown Docs are Dana Abendschein aka "Professor Dude," Curt Patty aka "Doctor ICU" and Diana Patty aka "Nurse Squiggles."

Dana Abendschein PhD, is a professor at Washington University School of Medicine in St. Louis, where he does vascular research and teaches several classes — including the first credit course on "The Medicine of Laughter" offered at any medical school in the country.

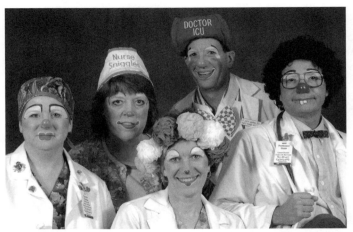

St. Louis Clown Docs are (from left) Jane "Dr. Tickles" Abendschein, Diana "Nurse Squiggles" Patty, Debbi "Bubbles the Scrub Nurse" Schwarz (seated) Curt "Doctor ICU" Patty and Dana "Professor Dude" Abendschein.

Dana and Jane teach all aspects of clowning including makeup, character development, and the use of clowning in hospitals and prisons.
To contact them or to learn about the Clown Docs program at St. Louis Children's Hospital, contact Jane Abendschein, 1401 Norman Place, Warson Woods, MO 63122, (314) 822-5315, libertyandbelle@aol.com

Curt and Diana Patty also teach all aspects of clowning. Contact them at P.O. Box 19722 St. Louis MO 63144, 314-962-3984
Email: clowngadgetstore@juno.com
Website: www.clowngadgetstore.com

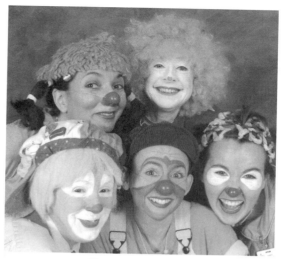

Clockwise from top left: Lucia "Nuula" Cino; Camilla "Posy" Gryski, Kate "Turtle" Keenan, Kathleen "Le Roux" Doko, Joan "Bunky" Barrington

Contact: Joan Barrington
Coordinator, Therapeutic
Clown Program, The Hospital
for Sick Children
Department of Child Life
555 University Avenue
Toronto, Ontario M5G 1X8
(416) 813-6629
joan.barrington@sickkids.ca

The Therapeutic Clown Program of The Hospital for Sick Children

"In the late 80's I was blessed with a dream and over the years, with the help of many dear friends, this dream has come to fruition," recalls Joan "Bunky" Barrington. "In 1993 Karen Ridd, aka Robo (the founder of the first Canadian Therapeutic Clown Program) together with myself established the first Therapeutic Clown Program in Ontario at The Hospital for Sick Children. Since its inception, the program has grown to five therapeutic clowns gently working their magic on five inpatient floors, two full days a week.

"Our therapeutic clowns are seasoned professionals with extensive backgrounds in areas such as theatre, clown, voice and movement, child development, holistic education and the expressive arts. The therapeutic clown truly comes from the 'inside out' and in each character we honour their unique spirit and magical self.

"I view love, warmth and a full expression of joy and wonderment as major components to the healing process and of being an effective and compassionate therapeutic clown.

"In therapeutic clowning there exists the three 'Cs'; *communication* which builds the trust, *connection* which opens the doors to healing and *compassion* that feeds the spirit. Through the relationship and intimacy, we can joyfully pass the control over to them and they will lead us. To move forward in life, hope is essential. The human spirit is powerful and these children have the capacity to live life to the fullest right up to the end. We are partners in the play, as we are partners in this life."

University Initiatives

Recent developments at two major universities are reinforcing the potential and value of therapeutic clowning in healing.

In one development, the first credit course in clowning is now being offered at a leading medical school—The Washington University School of Medicine in St. Louis.

In another development, an innovative initiative is underway at a major land-grant university, Penn State University, to explore applications of all the arts to health and healing issues.

Arts and Health Outreach Initiative (AHOI)
The Pennsylvania State University

This innovative, interdisciplinary initiative at The Pennsylvania State University, a leading land-grant university, is in the second year of a three year pilot project.

AHOI links the arts with a wide array of academic disciplines and external resources connected to personal and public health concerns. This allows AHOI to create coalitions that explore applications of the arts to personal health and healing, as well as to critical public health issues.

The initiative is supported by four principal Penn State partners— the Colleges of Arts and Architecture, Health and Human Development, and Medicine, and Penn State Outreach and Cooperative Extension.

AHOI embraces a broad definition of health, including not only personal health and healing, but also holistic community life and well-being.

Ermyn F. King, Coordinator

For more about the programs, conferences, exhibitions and other projects presented by AHOI, contact:
Arts and Health Outreach Initiative (AHOI)
Ermyn F. King, Coordinator
The Pennsylvania State University
3-D Keller Building
University Park, PA 16802
(814) 865-8230
Email: efk103@psu.edu

"To our knowledge, no other university has brought together as many diverse partners for the purpose of demonstrating and documenting the interrelationships between the arts and health.

"What universities have to offer is integration of teaching, research and service (and the outreach component of these core missions) in the arts and health."

Ermyn King, Coordinator,
Arts and Health Outreach Initiative
The Pennsylvania State University

Washington University School of Medicine offers course on "The Medicine of Laughter"

The Washington University School of Medicine is the first U.S. medical school to offer a credit course in clowning.

The credit selective course called "The Medicine of Laughter" has been offered for first year medical students since 2000. In the course, the medical students read and discuss literature describing the physiologic and psychological benefits of humor, and discuss how humor can play a positive role in the doctor/patient relationship.

The students also shadow the Clown Docs at St. Louis Children's Hospital to observe the effects of humor in the hospital setting. Students that choose to do so may participate in a "super-selective", in which they develop their own clown character.

Notes Professor Dana Abendschein, *(right)*, who teaches the course, "Our first goal is to not make students clowns, but to allow them to learn how to access humor to help themselves and their future patients."

For details on teaching of humor in medical school contact Dana Abendschein, Ph.D., Washington University School of Medicine, 660 South Euclid Box 8086, St. Louis, MO 63110, (314) 362-8925, dabendsc@im.wustl.edu

Hospital Clown Presenters

This list is not inclusive of every fine presenter. We offer it as a starting reference if you are seeking persons with extensive hospital clown experience, "best practice" knowledge and teaching experience.

Dana Abendschein   p. 68.
Jane Abendschein   p. 68.
Joe Barney (see below)
Joan Barrington   p. 69.
The Bumper "T" Caring Clowns p. 60.
Loretta DeAngelus   p. 62.
Carole Johnson   p. 64.
Susie Kleinwachter   p. 64.
Tammy Miller p. 82.
Debbie Nupp   p. 66.

Mary O'Brien   p. 63.
Curt Patty   p. 68.
Diana Patty   p. 68.
Desirae Payne p. 65.
Shobhana Schwebke   p. 67.
Richard Snowberg   p. 67.
Anita Thies p. 83.
Korey Thompson   p. 61.
Janet Tucker p. 80.
Patty Wooten   p. 9 & 76.

Joe Barney aka "Doc Geezer" (picture next page)
formerly clowned at Yale New Haven Children's Hospital
Contact him at: 129 Nutmeg Rd., Bridgeport, CT 06610 (203) 365-0571
Email: bamboozele@aol.com
Website: www.centerringproductions.com

Chapter 8
Your Future Journey

Hospital clowning is growing—in depth, training and impact around the world. Your future journey will build on work done by pioneering hospital clowns in recent years.

Growing Respect

Some noted therapeutic clown programs now are celebrating five and 10 years of service. Their years of professional service have generated greater acceptance of hospital clowning within the medical community.

Joan Barrington, Coordinator of the 10-year-old Therapeutic Clown Program at The Hospital for Sick Children in Toronto, Ontario, Canada observes:

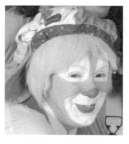

Joan as "Bunky"

"Therapeutic clowning at our hospital has become valued and respected by the health care team and parents alike.

"We are under the umbrella of the Child Life Department, are part of the multi-disciplinary team, go to Rounds when possible, take notes on all our interventions, keep stats and are accountable in every way as permanent part-time staff."

Korey Thompson, Artistic Director of Clowns for Children's Hospital of Wisconsin in Milwaukee, notes that, "now that we're in the fifth year of our program, we're more a part of the care giving team and that makes sense."

Role for Trained Volunteers

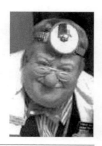

"I see hospital clowns being more widely accepted," agrees Joe "Doc Geezer" Barney, *(right)*, who formerly clowned at Yale New Haven Children's Hospital and now travels the country teaching hospital clowning. He adds, "I see more of a future role for trained volunteer groups."

Standards and Certification

In the United States, The Bumper "T" Caring Clowns are working with the Association for Applied and Therapeutic Humor and others to raise the bar on acceptable standards for hospital clowns and to develop a national certification procedure for hospital caring clowns.

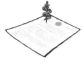

In Canada, Joan Barrington is working with a team to develop a curriculum with standards and procedures for Canadian therapeutic clown apprentices. In 1999, Joan became Co-Director of Therapeutic Clowns Canada, a not-for-profit organization that assists pediatric health care facilities in starting their programs.

The Future of the Healing Arts

Shobhana "Shobi Dobi" Schwebke believes that in time, more in the health care community "will value the caring clown's presence as a key to setting an essential environment for healing."[13]

As medical practices evolve, new doors may open for the healing humor of hospital clowns. Ermyn King, Coordinator of the Arts and Health Outreach Initiative at Penn State University observes that:

"The visionary Leland Kaiser speaks about the need for patients to have personal 'arts profiles' that will be factored into their healing regimen.

"Appropriate arts dosages including the art of healing humor, may be prescribed in a fashion hand-tailored to individual patients."

Ermyn King adds that it is not difficult to *"imagine healing arts centers incorporated into or attached to hospitals, permitting even discharged patients to continue their arts involvements to help maintain wellness and prevent symptom recurrence."*

In the meantime, hospital clown training programs are multiplying. The internet is linking hospital clowns everywhere. Clown trips throughout the world are becoming popular. Your future journey into hospital clowning can take you as far as you're willing to travel.

Some Parting Thoughts

"Only a life lived for others is worthwhile"--Albert Einstein

You May Never Know

*"Accept the reality
that you may never know
—you may never know
who is benefiting
from your entertainment
or presence.
You may never know
what impact you provide.
You may never know
what happens to some
of the individuals
that you encounter.
Finally, you may never know,
at the time of an encounter,
how this moment
will change your life
and stay with you forever."*
– Richard Snowberg

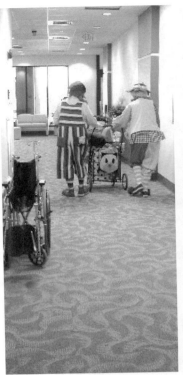

Betty "Dr. I See You" Hodgson
(left) and Peggy "Sunflower" Cole
finish rounds in State College, PA

How Do I Keep My Heart Open?

"I sit before the mirror, pasting this red nose on my face. It has become such a part of me, a nose I trust to help me open the door to a sick little boy's heart. I wonder if I will have the sensitivity and skill that is required to "be there" with his pain.

"I know the answers are all in my heart, but how do I keep my heart open in the face of his suffering? How can I keep it together and not become unglued?

"I need some wisdom greater than that inside of me. I know that I can be a channel, a vessel, an instrument of love and peace. I know that God will help me, if I only ask. But what does God know about clowning?

"And then I remember, this isn't about being a clown. It's about letting the love of God pour through me, while I'm dressed as a clown. The costume and make-up will get the little boy's attention, but the real healing power will come through my ability to love and accept, to forgive and surrender. I know I must Let Go and Let God." [14]   —Patty Wooten

Chapter 9
Resources

Our Top Recommendations:

The Hospital Clown Newsletter

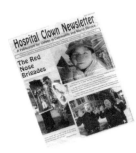

This excellent quarterly, international publication written and edited by "Shobi Dobi" reports the latest on hospital clowns, programs, props and ideas from around the world. Published quarterly for US $20 per year. Checks accepted. Contact: The Hospital Clown Newsletter, P.O. Box 8957, Emeryville, California 94662 (510) 420-1511 Fax (801) 751-6848 Email: ShobiDobi@hospitalclown.com Website: www.hospitalclown.com

The Hospital Clown: A Closer Look

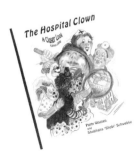

What Hospitals Need to Know About Clowns
What Clowns Need to Know about Hospitals

Published in 2000, this 195-page book is full of stories and pictures of hospital clown programs throughout the world. Authors: Shobi Dobi (above) and Patty Wooten. Order from Shobi at The Hospital Clown Newsletter (above) for $US20 plus $4 postage USA; $7 postage Canada.

The Caring Clowns: How Humor, Smiles and Laughter Overcome Pain, Suffering and Loneliness

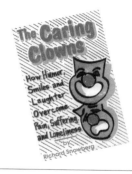

by Richard Snowberg
Order this classic soon while copies remain. Contact Richard Snowberg at Visual Magic, 1223 South 28th Street, LaCrosse, WI 54601 His email (at Clown Camp®) is snowberg.rich@uwlax.edu

The Lighter Side of Breast Cancer Recovery

Author: Tammy Miller, "Hugz the Clown." This book takes you down the path with a woman who has been there but it may not be the path most people follow. From surgeons equipped with clown noses to going through surgery wearing a feather boa, Tammy looks at this very serious topic with a lighthearted attitude and some words of encouragement for others facing a difficult journey. For information on this book's distribution, contact Tammy at 530 Hillside Avenue, State College, PA 16803 (814) 231-3001 Website: http://www.hugzandcompany.com/

Almost Home: Embracing The Magical Connection Between Positive Humor & Spirituality

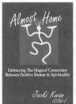

Author: Jacki Kwan, LCSW-C, Cameo Publications ISBN 0-9715739-1-3, 144 pages, $14.99 (USD) + S/H (March 2002) "For quite a while, my mission has been to heal the world one 'ha' at a time," says Jacki, a clinical social worker and creator of HA!HA!LOGY® Humor Therapy for Long-Term Care. "Now I realize the 'ahs' are just as important." Contact Jacki at jacki@hahalogy.com (301) 907-4610 PO Box 30769 Bethesda, MD 20824-0769 Website: www.hahalogy.com

Coming Soon: Schtick or Treat by Shobi Dobi. Great "schticks" for hospital clowns. Contact Shobi at address on previous page.

Coming Soon: Towel creations to make for patients

Debb Nupp plans to publish how to makes towels into dogs, swans, and more that you leave with the patient. See her address on p. 66.

More Great Books

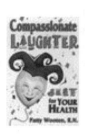

Compassionate Laughter 2nd ed. $15
Author: Patty Wooten This book looks at laughter for your body, mind and spirit.
Humor, Heart and Healing also by
Patty $10 Fun filled, laugh provoking quotes Both from Patty at Jest Press (831) 475-9570 Website: www.jesthealth.com Pwooten@jesthealth.com

More Great Resources

Laughter the Universal Language Author: Leslie Gibson
This is set up as a home study course and can provide nurses with 10 hours of continuing education credit. The cost for non-credit is $10.00 + $5.00 postage. The cost for the workbook WITH credit is $20.00 + $5.00 postage. Order from Leslie at laughaide@aol.com or call (727) 937-4746

Red clown noses for caring clown activities: For subscribers of The Hospital Clown newsletter only, contact Shobi Dobi (see p. 75.)

Clown Noses and Kazoos Hugz and Company (see p. 79.)

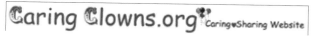

Website: http://www.caringclowns.org/ This website supports the caring clown movement by providing a virtual home for caring clowns. In addition to Caring Clown Forums, they have provided links to resources for ideas on juggling, magic, balloons, face painting, camps, workshops and anything else which might be of interest to caring clowns. It is sponsored by the Foundation for Therapeutic Clowning, PO Box 712, Carefree, Arizona 85377 (480) 488-4745

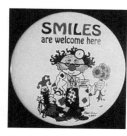

Smile Buttons and other resources from The Cancer Club

The Cancer Club provides humorous and helpful products for people with cancer. Books, audiocassettes, videotapes, PC software, custom jewelry and more. Subscribe to a quarterly newsletter and join The Cancer Club. Don't forget to laugh! TM Call: 1-800-586-9062
The Smile Button is $2
Website: www.cancerclub.com
Email: Christine@cancerclub.com   Christine K. Clifford, CSP CEO/ President The Cancer Club 6533 Limerick Drive Edina, MN 55439

"A shared gift of laughter is a priceless gift to the Spirit"
—Christine Clifford, President of The Cancer Club.

Clown Supplies

Center Ring Productions Hospital clown props and other supplies from Joe "Doc Geezer" Barney, 129 Nutmeg Rd., Bridgeport, CT 06610, (203) 365-0571 Email: bamboozele@aol.com
Website coming at http://www.centerringproductions.com

Charlie's Creative Comedy (Bruce Johnson)

 Bruce "Charlie" Johnson is an internationally known clown, family entertainer, instructor, author and artist. Through his company, Charlie's Creative Comedy, Bruce provides props and educational publications for clowns and other variety artists. His products are available only through mail order or at his dealer table when he is an instructor. We love his website with its free directions on making a napkin rose and great books such as "trick cartoons" that even those without artistic ability can learn to do at a patient's bedside. Contact Charlie's Creative Comedy, P.O.Box 82165, Kenmore, WA 98028-0165 Email: clownjuglr@aol.com Phone (425) 481-7143 Website: http://www.charliethejugglingclown.com/

 Clown City Supplies for clowns, magicians, puppeteers, clown ministers, and entertainers of all kinds. For a 280-page full color catalog (at no charge) call or email a request and they send it free of charge in the continental U.S. and Canada or download their catalog on-line. (860) 889-1000 phone & fax 509 Norwich Ave. Taftville, CT 06380
Email: clowncity@snet.net Website: http://www.clowncityonline.com/

Clown Gadget Store

 Specializing in clown props for hospitals and nursing homes Curt and Diana Patty (left), who clown with the St. Louis Clown Docs, have started this store specializing in hospital clowning as well as other comedy props, face paints, kazoos, bubble products, foam props and more.
"Hospital props should be made of latex free materials that are easy to clean. Please send us a note if you have a question to see if the prop you have chosen is recommended for hospital clowning. Our goal is to be a resource for humor therapy."
Their wide variety of props include a clown stethoscope, a "stool" sample and humor medical tests. Visit their on-line catalog at: www.clowngadgetsstore.com   Call or fax: (314) 962-3984; write: P.O. Box 19722, St. Louis, MO 63144 Email: clowngadgetstore@juno.com

---

Clown Supplies

Dewey's Good News Balloons Items of interest to hospital clowns include thumb tips, silks, rubber chickens, comedy props and books. Website: http://www.flash.net/~balloonz/ Email: balloonz@flash.net 1202 Wildwood Drive Deer Park, TX 77536-4079 (888) 894-6597

David Ginn Magic 370 Bay Grove Road, Loganville, GA 30052 (770) 466-8421 Great kidshow items. Email: ginnmagic@mindspring.com On line comedy magic catalog at: http://www.ginnmagic.com
Laughter Legacy Author: David Ginn. 1300 jokes, gags, one-liners, quips, and bits of comedy wisdom, 224 pages $25

HoBo Art Honey Leas and Bonita Hix create unique clothing, purses, quilts, pillows with your clown picture transferred on cloth, blouses and even checkbook covers. The purses can double as a small clown bag. Contact them at HoneyBonitaSew@aol.com (562) 690-0616

Handmade purse with pockets inside

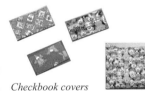

All-clown pillow and picture pillow of fall foliage trip

Checkbook covers

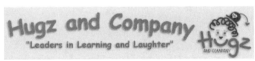

"Leaders in Learning and Laughter"

Hugz and Company
Tammy "Hugz" Miller offers clown noses, kazoos, novelty items and books including *The Lighter Side of Breast Cancer Recovery*. Her company provides workshops, training, and clowning, all emphasizing humor and creativity. 530 Hillside Avenue, State College, PA 16803 (814) 231-3001 Email: tammy@hugzandcompany.com Website: http://www.hugzandcompany.com/

Juggles Clown Props and Supplies
Lee "Juggles" Mullally 1817 SW 76th Terrace
Gainesville, FL 32607-3417
Website: ccjuggles@bellsouth.net
(352) 332-6092 Website coming soon

Susie "Pancakes" Kleinwachter
"Klein Time" Entertainment

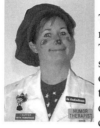

This full time clown, storyteller and public speaker sells many items geared for hospital and nursing home clowns. These include giant 16 inch band-aids; Dr. clown bag starter kit with props; squeakers, smiles on a stick, original badges and buttons, music, unique crazy hats, themed headbands, storytelling kits, "free B's," million dollar bills, little miracle cards, instructional audio casettes and much more.

Contact Susie Kleinwachter, Klein Time Entertainment, P.O. Box 700, Warrenville, IL 60555 Phone: (630) 393-7714 Email: FunE98@aol.com Website: http://www.KleinTime.com

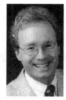

Samuel Patrick Smith SPS Magic & Publications

Great kid show items, magic, videos, audios, books.
SPS Publications P.O. Box 787 Eustis, Florida 32727
24-hour Order Line 1-800-810-0722
Website: http://www.spsmagic.com/

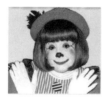

Carol Spaulding "Everyday's A Holiday"

Carol "Holiday" Spaulding is a professional clown, storyteller and costume designer. For hospital clowns, she offers original hats, vests, bows, bibs and storytelling supplies. Contact her at: 251 Cosworth Ct. Riva MD 21140 (410) 956-5275 Email: holidaytheclown@att.net Website: http://www.holiday-the-clown.com/

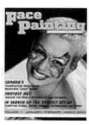

Silly Farm Products; Face Painting Magazine

Marcela "Mama Clown" Murad offers face paints, books, videos and supplies for clowns. Her international face painting magazine debuted in 2001. Contact Silly Farm Products, 2142 Tyler St., Hollywood, Florida 33020 (954) 923-6013 Website: http://www.sillyfarm.com/ Email: info@sillyfarm.com • orders@sillyfarm.com For her magazine: http://www.facepaintingmagazine.com/

Janet "Jelly Bean" Tucker 6334 New Hampshire Ave. Hammond, IN 46323 (219) 844-2858 Email: clowns.etc@poboxes.com Website: http://www.jellybean-clown.com

Magazines and Newsletters

Clowning Around published 10 times/year by the World Clown Association. Write P.O. Box 776236, Corona, CA 92877-1017 (800) 336-7922 Website: http://www.worldclownassociation.com/

Clowns Canada Quarterly News Clowns Canada is an organization of clowns, jugglers, magicians, face-painters, balloon artists and other entertainers. Most live in Canada, but there are members worldwide. Toll Free 1-877-654-6518 Website: http://www.clownscanada.com/

Face Painting International—See page 80.

Funny Paper, a Magazine for Family Entertainers. Write Chris Van Krieken, Suite 807, 80 Inverlochy Blvd., Thornhill, Ontario, Canada C3T 4P3, toll-free 1-866-235-5550 Website: http://www.funnypapermag.com/

Hospital Clown Newsletter— See page 75.

The New Calliope Published six times/year by Clowns of America International. Write P.O. Box Clown, Richeyville, PA 15358-0532, 1-888-52-Clown Website: http://www.coai.org/

Organizations

Association for Applied and Therapeutic Humor (AATH) 1951 W. Camelback Rd., Suite 445, Phoenix, AZ 85015 (602) 995-1454 Email: office@aath.org Website: http://www.aath.org/

The Society for the Arts in Healthcare 1632 U Street, NW, Washington, DC 20009 Phone: (202)299-9770 Fax: (202)299-9887 Email: mail@theSAH.org Website: www.theSAH.org

FOOTNOTES Section

1.Pg. 9: Patty Wooten, *The Hospital Clown Newsletter*, Vol. 4, 1999 and Wooten, Patty, *Compassionate Laughter*,
2.Pg. 9: Rev. George Burn in "Laughter Makes Good Medicine" by Anita Thies; *HORIZONS Magazine*, Presbyterian Church U.S.A., Jan.-Feb. 1997, p. 4
3.Pg. 11: Cousins, Norman, *Anatomy of an Illness.* .
4.Pg. 12: Richard Snowberg, *The Caring Clowns,*
5.Pg. 13: Richard Snowberg *The Caring Clowns,*
6.Pg. 18: Richard Snowberg, Clown Camp Notebook® Univ Wisconsin, LaCrosse
7.and 8 Pg. 25: Shobhana Schwebke Hospital Clown

Newsletter, Vol. 4, 1999
9.Pg. 31: Richard Snowberg, *The Caring Clowns*
10,Pg. 38: Centre Community Hospital, State College, PA. Manual for Pastoral Care Volunteers
11.Pg. 42: Janet "Jelly Bean" Tucker, Clown Alley 1982 issue
12,Pg. 43: Centre Community Hospital, State College, PA. Manual for Pastoral Care Volunteers
13Pg. 73: Shobhana Schwebke Hospital Clown Newsletter
14 Pg. 74: Compassionate Laughter and Hospital Clown Newsletter, Vol. 4, 1999

About the Authors and Illustrator

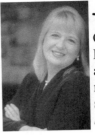

Tammy Miller is the owner of Hugz and Company Consulting in State College, Pennsylvania. Her company presents workshops on a variety of topics relating to humor, creativity, motivation, attitude, communication, presentation skills and clowning. She is the author of *The Lighter Side of Breast Cancer Recovery.*

Tammy is a Distinguished Toastmaster, the highest educational and leadership distinction of Toastmasters International. A co-founder and vice president of The Happy Valley Alley of the World Clown Association, Tammy traveled as an invited guest to Gabrovo, Bulgaria in 2002 to clown and instruct workshops for the International House of Humour. She holds an M.A. degree from Penn State University. Tammy may be reached at 530 Hillside Avenue, State College, PA 16803 (814) 231-3001 Email: tammy@hugzandcompany.com
Website: http://www.hugzandcompany.com/

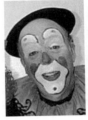

Bill Moore started drawing his own adventure strips at a very young age, stealing concepts from all the popular action comics of the 1940s. On his way to becoming a world renowned cartoonist he got side tracked into the ministry as a Presbyterian pastor. He says he has a lot in common with Jonah, who never made it to Tarshish. Bill has clowned at state schools, hospitals, nursing homes, and special events. He began clowning in the 1970s and named his clown in the 1990s ("Mo", short for the Greek word moros, which means fool, as in Fool for

Christ). Since retiring as a pastor in the year 2000, Bill and his wife Carol have celebrated the arrival of their granddaughter Brooke Hart.*(above)* Bill's sketches appear in the newsletter of the creative ministries organization Cheer Leaders for Christ.

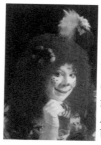

Kathy Piatt has been clowning around for over 20 years as "Popcorn." Born in Edmonton, Alberta, Canada, she was introduced to the art of clowning by her father at an early age and has been thankful ever since. She has studied in Canada and abroad—receiving a marketing degree from the University of Alberta, Sophia University in Tokyo and Penn State University. Kathy is a co-founder and past president of the Happy Valley Alley of the World Clown Association in State College, PA where she lives with her husband John and children Sean and Tavrie. She currently is studying to be a certified therapeutic massage therapist at the Mount Nittany Institute of Health. Special thanks to her parents-Bud and Laverna, and all the clowns she has met on and off the roads of Clown Camps ® along the way. Kathy may be reached at 114 Brandywine Drive, State College, PA 16801 (814) 234-1849 Email: jpiatt@geisinger.edu

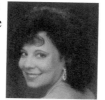

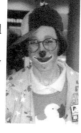

Anita Thies heard God's call into clowning in the early 1980s after receiving healing from a major depression. She has clowned in hospitals as "Dr. Duck" and in churches as "Toot." She attended Clown Camp ® at the University of Wisconsin LaCrosse in 1996 on a Mark Anthony Scholarship and was invited back to teach there in 2000 and 2003. A co-founder and past president of the Happy Valley Alley of the World Clown Association, she teaches nationally on caring clowning, clown ministry and the role of humor in healing.

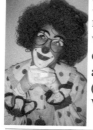

Her major focus currently is leading the creative ministries organization Cheer Leaders for Christ where she serves as president and editor of the quarterly national newsletter. Anita may be reached at 761 Cornwall Rd., State College, PA 16803 (814) 237-9466 Email: anitathies@yahoo.com Website: http://www.geocities.com/toot_the_clown/

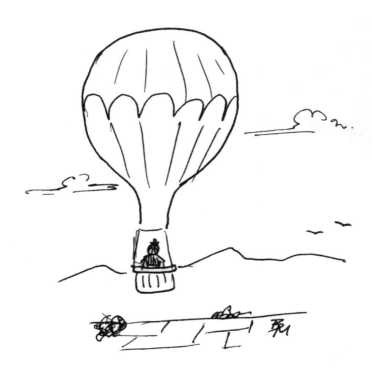

Have a Joyful Journey!

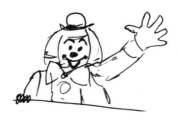

For more copies of this book:
Lighthearted Press
761 Cornwall Rd. State College, PA 16803
Email: joyfuljourneyclowning@yahoo.com
Call Anita Thies (814) 237-9466 (home)
Or email Anita at: anitathies@yahoo.com
http://www.geocities.com/lightheartedpress/index.html